Overcoming Common Problems

LEARNING TO LIVE WITH MULTIPLE SCLEROSIS

Dr Robert Povey, Robin Dowie
and Gillian Prett

Foreword by Professor Bryan Matthews
Illustrations by Keith Lovet Watson

sheldon PRESS

First published in 1981 by the Multiple Sclerosis
Society of Great Britain and Northern Ireland

Revised edition published in Great Britain in 1986
by Sheldon Press, SPCK, Marylebone Road, London NW1 4DU

Fourth impression 1992
Revised edition 1997

British Library Cataloguing in Publication Data
A catalogue record for this book is available from the British Library
ISBN 0–85969–760–6

Typeset by Deltatype Ltd, Birkenhead, Merseyside
Printed in Great Britain by Biddles Ltd, Guildford and King's Lynn

Contents

Foreword

People with multiple sclerosis and their families are in great need of information, first of all about the strange disease that has entered their life and caused more or less profound changes. Just as important is the need to know how best to cope with the many problems of everyday life that inevitably arise. The authors of this book have wisely based their advice on answers provided by multiple sclerosis sufferers themselves and those who help them to maintain their independence. In this context practical wisdom is worth far more than medical knowledge. I have no doubt that those in need who read this book will derive much comfort and support.

Bryan Matthews
Emeritus Professor of Clinical Neurology
University of Oxford

Acknowledgements

The inspiration for this book came from the members of the Canterbury and District Branch of the Multiple Sclerosis Society. Their warmth and spontaneity of friendship showed that multiple sclerosis was not to be feared but that the problems of living with it could be better understood. They gave their time and encouragement by preparing case histories about themselves and talking in groups about ways of coping with day-to-day tasks.

Marilyn Povey prepared the framework for the case histories. Then, drawing on her personal experience as a sufferer and her professional knowledge as an occupational therapist, she has offered ideas and advice at every stage in the preparation of the first and later editions of the book. Helpful comments on the earlier editions were received from Dr Marion Hildick-Smith, Professor Michael Warren, Joan Warren, Professor Michael Drake, Gill Williams and John Walford. Secretarial assistance was given by Kathleen Horton and Joan Robson. Valuable help with later revisions has been given by Dr Stephen Pollock, Sue Cover, Caroline Clarke and Peter Cardy, Chief Executive of the MS Society, who supplied most of the text for Chapter 7.

We are grateful for the help of all these people and for the encouragement of others who read the first draft of the book.

Preface

The first edition of this book was welcomed most enthusiastically by people with MS and their families, and since then thousands of copies have been sold in aid of the Canterbury and District branch of the MS Society. This new, third, edition has been extensively revised and rewritten. It includes a discussion of important new research developments on the nature of MS and its treatment (Chapter 2); a new chapter on exercise and diet (Chapter 6); a revised chapter on the MS Society (Chapter 7); and an updated section on benefits and allowances (Chapter 8). The remainder of the text has also been revised where necessary to take account of current developments in the management of MS.

We hope that the new edition will continue to prove helpful to MS sufferers and their families as well as to doctors, nurses, social workers, health visitors, physiotherapists, occupational therapists – in fact to anyone who cares for the disabled in a hospital or community setting.

1

The doctor's dilemma

Multiple sclerosis is a strange disorder. It doesn't have any really clear-cut symptoms in its early stages and it is very difficult to predict the likely course of the disease over a number of years. The problems experienced by one MS sufferer may be quite unlike those experienced by another. One person may show just a slow loss of mobility, gradually finding walking much more difficult, whereas another person might be confined to a wheelchair for six months completely unable to walk and then be apparently fighting fit for another ten years or more. In these circumstances the doctor is faced with some difficult decisions. The guidelines for action are much less clear than they would be in the case of more straightforward ailments such as measles or mumps.

Diagnosis

The immediate problem confronting the doctor is that of making an accurate diagnosis. The first sign of MS may be something which can appear at times in healthy people such as an occasional numbness or feeling of pins and needles in the fingers or toes, or a slight and temporary disturbance of vision. Quite often such symptoms appear only fleetingly and it would be foolish for a doctor to jump to firm diagnostic conclusions on such flimsy evidence. Over a period of time, however, other symptoms may appear, often in different parts of the body, and these spasmodic episodes come to form a more coherent picture. It is then that one hopes that the general practitioner will play the 'detective' role and begin to piece together a few bits of the jigsaw. At this stage it is likely that the patient will be referred to the hospital consultant. In some cases, of course, the GP doesn't suspect the existence of MS at all. The symptoms being treated may appear, for example, as minor complications of quite common complaints. Thus the tendency of MS patients to trip up on the corners of carpets or uneven pavements in the early stages of the disease may result in sprained ankles or broken bones which do not respond to treatment in the normal way. In such situations it may be the orthopaedic consultant at the hospital rather than the GP who suspects the existence of MS. The patient would then quite properly be referred to a more appropriate consultant – the neurologist.

Telling the patient

The diagnosis of neurological disease is an intricate and often time-consuming affair and even when the consultant has arrived at a diagnosis of MS the patient is sometimes not told that he or she has the disease. In some instances patients are sent away to contend with the continuing anxiety caused by their unexplained symptoms. To the layperson this seems a strange piece of behaviour by the medical profession, but non-disclosure of the diagnosis to the patient used to be a very widespread practice. What then are the reasons for this particular approach?

In the first place, the neurologist may not be completely certain about the diagnosis since the symptoms may be insufficiently clear. To tell a patient that he or she is suffering from a disabling disease when the neurologist is not quite certain about the diagnosis would obviously be wrong. Some form of follow-up examination is usually most appropriate in such circumstances. If, on the other hand, the neurologist is clear that the patient has MS, then why should this diagnosis be concealed? The medical answer advanced by those neurologists who have supported the 'non-disclosure' approach seems to be that it is always possible that the symptoms which the patient is currently experiencing might disappear (in other words, the patient might have a 'remission'), and there may be a period of several months or years in which the patient is symptom-free. In these circumstances it would be better that the patient should not be worried unnecessarily about the possible long-term consequences of the disease. One MS sufferer, for example, had a ten-year remission in between the first symptoms appearing and their reappearance. The first symptoms of pins and needles, turning over an ankle and light-headedness lasted on and off for about a year and then apparently disappeared for the next ten! During those ten years she had a family, a part-time job, went cycling and dealt adequately with all the day-to-day chores of a housewife. Her own comment is: 'I'm glad I didn't know what exactly was wrong with me, as I might have kept worrying about when it would return.' This is the sort of case which provides some support for the medical practice of 'non-disclosure'.

However, many doctors and perhaps the majority of MS sufferers now believe that after a *firm* diagnosis has been made and the symptoms have become increasingly disabling then it is time for the doctor to take the patient into his or her confidence. Indeed, there is evidence to suggest that failure to tell the patient can sometimes lead to distressing consequences. Thus one finds examples of MS sufferers finding out about their illness in a roundabout way: 'Doctors told me it was paraesthesia. This was over several years and many attacks. Multiple sclerosis was mentioned only when I was advised to apply for a disability allowance . . . Finding it out only confirmed my suspicions. I resented being kept in the dark.' 'I was not told I had MS. I found out when I was rushed into hospital with peritonitis following an ectopic pregnancy. I overheard a nurse reading out my doctor's letter.'

Clearly, the discovery of MS by such roundabout routes is likely to be far more devastating in its effects than the discovery in the GP's surgery or the hospital clinic. Although it is difficult to generalise, the experience of MS sufferers does suggest that if the symptoms are well established, 'being told' by the doctor can be a positive aid to the patient's adjustment. As one MS sufferer has said: 'It's my body and my life and I ought to have the right to know what's happening to them so that I can make an appropriate adjustment to the situation.' Indeed, the person with MS often needs to have the aid of a diagnosis in order to make sense of the symptoms which still persist and cause anxiety despite the doctor's reassurance. Many MS sufferers in our survey drew attention to the sense of relief they have experienced at knowing what is wrong with them. They have been wondering whether they are suffering from brain tumours, cancer or mental illness. When they are told about MS the 'jigsaw pieces begin to fit together'. They can make sense of their symptoms and begin to adjust to their condition.

This adjustment is also something which can only be accomplished adequately if MS patients are told about the disease. In the past the patient's relatives have sometimes been told without telling the patient, but nowadays it is felt that this is usually an unnecessary burden to cast on the relatives. It increases anxiety without offering the possibility of constructive adjustment on the part of the whole family.

The doctor is certainly placed in a dilemma and there is no simple rule which can be applied in all cases. Doctors now believe, however, that in the past too many MS patients have been kept in the dark unnecessarily and given insufficient opportunity to come to terms with their disease.[1] Professor Bauer, for example, claims that it is important 'to provide the worried patients with more complete and truthful information . . . An evasive answer may cause many patients to worry even more, because they conclude that the doctor does not know what the disease is, or that his diagnosis implies such a bad prognosis, that the doctor does not dare to reveal the whole truth.' It is clear that sensitive judgement is required in relation to the treatment of patients as individuals. The doctor should, therefore, 'set aside time to convey to the patient and his family correct information about the disease and its consequences. The aim should be to encourage them not to lose their confidence and to give them a reasonable hope of being able to live with their disease.'

2

Some information about the disease

Once people have been told that they have multiple sclerosis (disseminated sclerosis as it used to be called), then it is likely that they will be anxious to know more about the disease and why they should have contracted it. Unfortunately, multiple sclerosis is still not fully understood by doctors and medical scientists, even though it was identified as a distinct disease by Charcot in Paris in 1868. This chapter provides a brief summary of what is known about the disease and those who suffer from it.[1] If it seems rather technical it is because the disease process itself is complex.

Who are the sufferers?

In terms of the sex and age of newly diagnosed persons, most recent surveys agree that multiple sclerosis attacks women more frequently than men (by a ratio of about three to two) and on average at a slightly earlier age. For both sexes the risk of first developing symptoms rises steeply from early adolescence, reaching a peak in the early thirties. The risk then falls away with increasing age.

MS sufferers and their families may feel anxious about whether the disease is inherited. There does not seem to be any *direct* inheritance, because research on identical twins has shown that when one identical twin is affected it doesn't necessarily follow that the other twin will also have MS. In fact, in a recent survey of the incidence of MS in twins in the British Isles the disease was clinically identified as 'definitely' or 'probably' present in *both* identical twins in only about 20% of cases.[2] If MS was caused by direct inheritance both twins would invariably suffer from the disease since identical twins share virtually identical genes. However, MS does occur more often among the close relatives of those with the disease than in the general population (i.e. there is a 'familial tendency'), which may be due partly to genetic factors and partly to exposure of the families to a common environmental influence. The occurrence is highest in identical twins, considerably lower in non-identical twins (about 3% in the British Isles study), and decreasing in incidence as the degree of relationship becomes more distant. In general, MS in brothers and sisters tends to be more common than in parents and children. But it must be stressed that it is still very uncommon even among relatives, and that MS is not a contagious or infectious disease and cannot be caught through contact with someone who has it.

Anyone who has dealings with multiple sclerosis sufferers quickly realises that the course and severity of the disease varies greatly between individuals. At one extreme MS can cause severe disabilities in a previously healthy adult; at the other extreme it may have been present but undetected and the person may have lived to a ripe old age without suffering from any really disabling symptoms. In about one-tenth of cases the disorder is progressive from the start although with fluctuations. This is often referred to as 'primary progressive MS'. But the majority of sufferers have what is called 'relapsing-remitting' MS, with a history of relapses separated by stable periods (remissions) which can last for months or years. Sometimes, after several years, the remission may stop and the person may become progressively more disabled (this may be referred to as 'secondary progressive MS'). However, as we have already noted, the pattern of the disease varies markedly between individuals *whatever type of MS is involved*. Some studies have shown that in about a quarter of cases the disease is benign and the sufferer has a normal life span with relatively little disability for ten or even twenty years (or more) after the initial appearance of the symptoms. In general, it seems that the degree of disability experienced five years after the first symptoms occur is a good index for the future. If a sufferer has only mild disability at five years then the disease is likely to remain mild, although there will be exceptional cases. Other predictors of the likely progression of the disease are the type and frequency of relapses and the extent of recovery. If relapses are generally infrequent, however, or predominantly involve the optic nerve (such as temporary blurring of vision) or sensory pathways (such as tingling sensations in the limbs), then the outlook on the whole is optimistic.

Sufferers learn to cope with set-backs without necessarily going to see their family doctor.

The general health record of many sufferers is about the same as that of people without MS. In our branch of the MS Society, people who miss an outing or meeting because of ill-health are nearly as likely to be able-bodied members as MS sufferers, and the reasons tend to be common ailments such as coughs and colds rather than the disease itself. In the past, it has been shown that patients with multiple sclerosis tend to consult their doctor about problems caused by the disease far less frequently than patients with other chronic disorders such as bronchitis, asthma, arthritis and Parkinson's disease (in the older age groups).[3] One reason for this may be that until recently there has been only a limited range of treatments for multiple sclerosis relapses. However, with current developments in steroid and other drug treatments (discussed later in the chapter), patients with MS should begin to feel increasingly confident about the possibility of obtaining some form of medical treatment for their condition.

Occasionally the newspapers or television carry stories about someone dying from multiple sclerosis. These can give a misleading impression about the number of deaths caused by the disease. Only a tiny proportion of sufferers die from MS. It is much more likely for sufferers to die from common disorders such as respiratory infections, heart conditions or simply old age!

What is multiple sclerosis?

The disease affects the nerves in the central nervous system, that is, in the brain and spinal cord. (It is not a mental disorder.) The nerves consist of bundles of microscopic nerve fibres, and wrapping each fibre is a chemical sheath known as the myelin sheath. It is rather like the insulation protecting a telephone cable. In MS some powerful agent attacks the myelin sheath and it becomes inflamed. Sometimes this inflammation can die down without doing any permanent damage, but if the attack continues then the myelin sheath is destroyed, leaving lesions (plaques of scar tissue). Unfortunately, this scar tissue does not function as normal nerve tissue, and as a result many of the millions of fibres which run through the spinal cord fail to carry their messages clearly. The end result of this failure in the conduction of nerve messages is that various parts of the body cease to work properly.

It is thought that when somebody experiences his or her first symptoms, such as temporary loss of vision or a weakness in one or more limbs, there may be only one single plaque causing symptoms. When the symptoms recur, especially if they are in a different part of the body, the doctors can be more certain that plaques have formed in more than one area; that is to say, they are multiple. There are sufferers, however, whose symptoms affect two or more parts of the body from the start. There is no specific test widely available to diagnose multiple sclerosis, a situation which applies to many disorders of the nervous system and to other illnesses. When diagnosing two or more lesion sites, doctors have had to depend on the way patients have described and demonstrated their symptoms, which often include feelings of excessive fatigue. However, a number of techniques have been developed which help to make the diagnosis more accurate.

One of the most recent advances has been the development of magnetic resonance imaging (MRI), which is a safe radiological imaging technique involving the use of a magnetic field and radio waves. It enables doctors to identify lesions in the brain which were undetectable by other techniques. With MRI there is no risk of building up a dangerous dosage of radiation as there is with X-rays, so it can be used over and over again to assess patients' progress.

Although the MRI technique is important, it can sometimes be misleading and it must be stressed that there are a variety of other tests used in the diagnosis of MS, the tests selected for use in individual cases depending on the nature of the case and the resources available. Thus, in addition to MRI, another diagnostic scanning device often used in MS is the computerized assisted tomography (more commonly known as a CT or CAT scan). A number of neurophysiological tests (such as visual, auditory or somatosensory evoked responses) may also be used, and a sample of the cerebro-spinal fluid obtained for analysis by means of a lumbar puncture. Not all these tests will be necessary in each individual case, of course, and all the test results have to be interpreted in the light of the clinical evidence together with the patients' own accounts of their symptoms.

What causes multiple sclerosis?

Doctors and research scientists continue to be baffled about the cause of multiple sclerosis. The extensive research programmes throughout the world have not found out what causes the plaques to form nor why it happens in certain individuals. Since multiple sclerosis occurs exclusively in humans it has not been possible to look for clues from animal studies, although related animal diseases such as scrapie in sheep have been examined.

Studies of populations (epidemiological studies) show some striking trends in the geographical distribution of MS, and this evidence has encouraged researchers to look for the possibility of a common environmental agent as a factor in causing the disease. Amongst the most consistent findings from population studies are that the disease is especially common in temperate climates but rare in the tropics; it is found most frequently in white populations; and its incidence tends to increase as the distance from the equator increases. However, there are some notable exceptions to these general trends which indicate that factors such as the 'latitude effect' cannot provide the whole story. For example, according to the 'distance from the equator' argument, MS ought to be relatively common in Japan. In fact, it is comparatively rare in that country, although when it does appear it manifests itself in a particularly severe form of the disease. In terms of world-wide distribution, the high risk areas in the northern hemisphere tend to be the British Isles and northern and central Europe, together with Iceland, Canada and the northern states of the USA. In the southern hemisphere the high risk zone covers New Zealand, southern Australia and Tasmania. Studies have also shown that people who live in high risk areas in early life and then migrate to a low risk area still have a relatively high susceptibility to the disease.

It is estimated that in Great Britain at least 100 persons in 100,000 suffer from MS. But recent evidence suggests that this may underestimate the prevalence of MS. For example, in the London Borough of Sutton a survey of the social services department, the local branch of the MS Society, general practitioners, hospital departments, community nurses and other sources gave an overall prevalence figure of 115 per 100,000.[4] Similarly, prevalence rates of 117 per 100,000 have been found in south-east Wales and 153 in rural Suffolk; and according to General Practice records, the overall rate for England and Wales appears to be about 1 in 800 of the population and 1 in 600 in Scotland. Even higher rates than these are found in certain areas in the north. For example, in north-east Scotland a prevalence rate of 178 per 100,000 people has been found, and in the Orkney and Shetland islands the combined figure in a 1983 survey was well over 200 per 100,000 (i.e. more than 1 in 500).[5]

Other epidemiological evidence could suggest a familial factor even though MS is not directly inherited. For instance, we have already seen that the overall risk of getting MS in Japan is very much lower than would be expected from its latitude, and the Japanese still appear to have a low risk of developing the disease no matter where in the world they are born or live.

The population-based evidence has provided 'signposts' to valuable laboratory-based investigations. Just as everyone has a blood group so too we have tissue groups, and in the early 1970s it was discovered that MS occurs more frequently in certain tissue groups than in others. Research workers then began to identify the genes which determine tissue groups and since that time numerous gene types have been examined as possible candidates for conferring susceptibility to MS. Of these 'markers of susceptibility', as they are called, researchers appear to have identified certain clear genetic markers associated with the development of MS in northern European countries, but in other countries (e.g. Sardinia) different associations have been found. Scientists such as Professor Alastair Compston and his co-researchers at the University of Cambridge Neurology Unit are currently studying these important genetic markers. It appears from their research so far that there are likely to be a number of different genetic factors associated with MS, and that the chances of developing the disease are linked to ethnic background. In particular, it appears that MS is most common where the frequency of northern European genes is high.

It seems, therefore, that genetic factors are likely to play an important part in the development of MS and, according to Professor Compston and his co-researchers, the balance of evidence 'favours an interplay between genetic susceptibility and an environmental trigger'.[6] The evidence from migrant studies (i.e. studies of people who have moved from one country to another) emphasizes the importance of this interplay between nature and nurture in the development of MS. According to a recent study by Gale and Martyn at the University of Southampton's MRC Environmental Epidemiology Unit,[7] migrants moving from a country where the disease is common to one where it is rarer show a *decrease* in the incidence of the disease, indicating an influence of the new environment. On the other hand, as we have already seen with the Japanese, people moving from low to high risk areas tend to retain their low risk status, showing the effects of genetic factors. However, the subtlety of the interactions can be seen by the fact that children born *after* their parents' migration sometimes tend to have a risk level which approaches that of their adopted country. This is especially true of West Indian, Indian and African immigrants in the UK, but much less evident in orientals who have migrated to the USA.

In general, these findings are consistent with the view that both genetic and environmental factors play a part in the development of MS, and it appears from studies which have looked at the effect of age at migration that a person's risk of developing MS is largely established by the age of 20. The evidence also supports the hypothesis that there may be some sort of environmental agent, such as a virus, which triggers the disease process, resulting in demyelination in the central nervous system and the consequent formation of plaques. Over the years many viruses have been suggested as possible triggers, and there has been particular interest in late-onset measles. There have been several research reports indicating that the concentration of antibodies to measles is greater than expected in people with MS, but so far the research evidence is insufficiently clear-cut to implicate measles directly as a relevant trigger virus. However, this research has strengthened the speculation that the trigger may be some sort of *delayed* exposure to a common infectious agent; and in fact there is some indication that people who develop MS tend to have suffered from the common childhood infections such as measles, mumps and rubella rather later than usual.

One virus which may fit into this picture is the Epstein-Barr virus, which causes infectious mononucleosis (more commonly known as glandular fever). In some countries (e.g. Denmark) centralised records are kept of blood tests for the Epstein-Barr virus, and it has been possible to compare these with the records of patients who have developed MS. When these comparisons were made in one Danish study it was found that people infected with the Epstein-Barr virus beyond the early years of childhood had nearly a 3-fold increase in their risk of developing MS. However, despite these interesting findings much more research is required before firm conclusions can be drawn about the possible role of the Epstein-Barr virus in MS.

Another problem with the virus hypothesis is that there is as yet no clear indication as to how a particular virus could trigger the demyelination process. Amongst the most promising theories is one which argues that in some people (who may have similar genetic factors) a virus could be triggering the auto-immune responses that protect the body from infection, and it is suggested that these responses themselves may cause the demyelination (the formation of the plaques).[8] In this way the body's immune responses (in particular the white blood cells called T-lymphocytes, which are designed to attack and destroy foreign invaders such as germs) actually begin to reject and destroy healthy parts of the body, such as myelin. This theory is supported by evidence from animal studies involving a disease called experimental allergic encephalomyelitis (EAE), which resembles MS in certain respects. Much research has yet to be done in this field, but if a specific viral agent can be identified it might be possible to develop a vaccine against MS, just as the measles and poliomyelitis vaccines were produced.

Treatment in MS

Ideally, research into the cause of MS would already have established the exact nature of the process involved in demyelination, so that treatment could now be developed to stop the process or, better still, reverse it by stimulating remyelination (i.e. the replacement of the damaged sheaths with new myelin). Unfortunately, we have not yet reached that position, but scientists are beginning to discover some important clues about the conditions under which remyelination might take place. It is known, for example, that during normal development the cells which produce myelin (called oligodendrocytes) grow from oligodendrocyte precursors (OPs), and scientists at the Cambridge Centre for Brain Repair, working with MS-like damage in rats, have discovered that it is possible, by transplanting OPs, to achieve remyelination of areas of the spinal cord.[9] The Cambridge team feels that it should be possible, eventually, to transplant human OP cells into people with MS to stimulate remyelination. There is a long way still to go, but with a 'massive funding' commitment from the MS Society there is every hope that we will have the means of repairing the damage to the brain and spinal cord in MS within the foreseeable future. Meanwhile, an effective treatment for the symptoms in MS could be developed even before the exact nature of the disease process has been established, and many of the treatment approaches discussed in this chapter have proceeded along these lines.

Problems evaluating treatment in MS

There are considerable difficulties involved in assessing the effectiveness of potential treatments in MS, and it is all too easy to raise people's hopes of new 'miracle cures' which have apparently worked for one or two individuals only to be found wanting when they have been rigorously tested in large-scale clinical trials. One particular difficulty in MS is that spontaneous remissions can occur without any clear cause, and improvements in symptoms are not always related to specific treatments or events so much as to the natural course of the disease. For example, relapses tend to occur less frequently as part of the natural progress of the disease, and so it is sometimes difficult to evaluate at the end of a treatment programme what constitutes *genuine* improvement based on the effects of the treatment and what are changes in the natural pattern of the disease over time. Where potential treatments seem to have been of benefit to a handful of individual MS sufferers, however, it is sensible for these to be tested more fully. In the first place, it would be usual to test a treatment approach in a pilot study using a small group of perhaps 10–20 subjects; and then, if the results are encouraging, to subject it to further rigorous analysis in a large-scale, scientifically controlled trial such as that described below in relation to beta interferon. Smaller-scale clinical trials are currently being carried out by the pharmaceutical firm Scotia on a possible combined drug treatment which has recently (1995) received considerable publicity.[10] It is very important, however, to await the results of the relevant controlled clinical trials before such experimental medication is considered for general use in the treatment of MS.

Antiviral treatment

If it does turn out to be the case that MS is triggered by a virus, then some form of antiviral treatment is likely to play an important part in treatment. For a long time little progress was made in the effort to find possible antiviral agents, but clinical trials with a drug based on the substance beta interferon have provided a more encouraging picture. Interferon is a protein that is produced naturally in our bodies by cells that have been infected by a virus, and it appears to act as one of the body's defence mechanisms against such infection. There are three types of interferon, namely alpha, beta and gamma, and they all have effects on our immune system in addition to helping protect the body from viruses and diseases, such as cancer, in which cells multiply in an uncontrolled manner. There are also different forms of beta interferon, and research has been carried out on substances identified as beta interferon 1a and beta interferon 1b. Neither offers a cure for the underlying disease process, but both appear to have potential for reducing the rate of relapse in MS patients. Apart from its antiviral effects, beta interferon has the added advantage of appearing to interfere with some of the signals the body sends to cells of the immune system which, in MS, seem programmed to attack healthy nerve cells. A drug called Betaferon, based on beta interferon 1b and produced by genetic engineering, received a UK licence in December 1995 for the treatment of relapsing-remitting MS, and other interferon products are expected to receive licences in due course.

The pioneering work on beta interferon 1b has been carried out by research workers in Canada and the USA.[11] Beta interferon 1b was administered by injection in two dose strengths to over 200 patients suffering from relapsing-remitting MS (half receiving the stronger dose and half the weaker). Their progress was then compared with over 100 comparable MS patients who formed the control group and who were given a placebo (i.e. they were administered injections which did not contain any form of medication). The patients were assigned to the treatment group or control group at random, and the experiment was designed as a double blind trial (i.e. to prevent any unintentional bias interfering with the results, neither medical staff nor patients knew to which group they had been assigned). The study extended over a total period of 5 years, but the effects of the treatment were clearly apparent in the early part of the study and these were maintained throughout. The authors report, for example, that after three years of treatment 'the study showed an approximately one-third reduction in the frequency of exacerbations and a 50 per cent reduction in severe exacerbations' (i.e. in the high-dose treatment group compared with the placebo group). There was also a significant difference in the rate of lesion progression, as detected by MRI scan, between the high-dose group and the controls, the rate of active lesions in the high-dose group showing clear reductions compared with the placebo group in which lesions tended to *increase* over the period of the study.[12] No major side effects were apparent, although it was quite common for patients to suffer some irritation at the site of the injection, and a few people suffered from bouts of depression. Something like a third of patients on the high-dose drug also developed antibodies to beta interferon in the first two years of the study, which resulted in the treatment becoming less effective for those patients compared with patients who did not develop such antibodies. Another quite common side effect at the beginning of treatment was the development of flu-like symptoms, but in most cases these disappeared after a few weeks.

Initially Betaferon will be available in the UK only for MS sufferers with the relapsing-remitting form of the disease, since this is the only group of patients on which we so far have evidence of the effects of the drug. However, research is in progress to examine what effect interferon substances have on MS sufferers with the progressive form of the disease; and a drug, Avonex (based on beta interferon 1a), which may help to reduce both relapse rate and *progression of disability* in MS, is already in production.[13] As far as Betaferon is concerned, it is likely that patients who satisfy the relapsing-remitting criteria will need to be referred by the GP to a consultant neurologist, in order that suitability for treatment can be confirmed. If a patient is accepted for treatment the consultant neurologist will arrange for the drug to be prescribed; patients will probably be taught how to inject themselves with the drug and arrangements will be made for the progress of the patient's MS to be monitored.[14] Although drugs based on interferon do not offer a *cure* for MS, their introduction as a form of treatment for controlling the exacerbation rate in some forms of MS is an exciting development, and the continuation of research in this field raises the possibility of even more effective treatments in future.

Immunosuppression

On the basis of the theory that MS is an auto-immune disease in which the body's own defence system is attacking the myelin, several studies have focused on the use of drugs which help to suppress the immune reactions (i.e. immunosuppressant drugs). Several drugs have been tried, sometimes in combination with steroids, but without conspicuous success. Some improvements in MS have been evident in a few studies, but often with the use of very large toxic doses and at the expense of unpleasant side effects. Greater success has been achieved recently, however, with the drug cladribine, which regulates the level of white blood cells in the blood. This drug appears to have a beneficial influence on the course of progressive MS, and to result in a decrease in the frequency of relapses in the relapsing-remitting form of the disease. Azathioprine may also have a limited role to play in the treatment of progressive MS.

Steroid treatments

These treatments were introduced on the pragmatic grounds that they had been found to be valuable in promoting recovery in other diseases and, in particular, in another demyelinating disease called post-infective encephalomyelitis. The term 'steroids' tends to be used to cover cortisone-based preparations such as prednisolone and prednisone, and also a pituitary gland preparation known as ACTH. This latter preparation is not strictly speaking a steroid itself, but it stimulates the production of steroids, including cortisone, by the adrenal gland. As usual in evaluating treatments in MS, it is difficult to judge the benefits of the drugs since because they are not usually given until a relapse occurs, there is no way of knowing if the recovery is the result of the drug or just the natural course of the disease. But there is sufficient evidence from controlled trials and from clinical experience to accept steroids as a useful form of treatment for relapses in MS, and one which is likely to provide relatively swift (even if sometimes only temporary) benefit. Steroids are only recommended for use on a short-term basis, however, since they can have side effects and become less effective over time. In general, ACTH has tended to provide the mainstay of steroid therapy, but there is some evidence that a five-day course of methylprednisolone, administered intravenously, may be more effective.[15] This does, however, involve the patient's admission to hospital for the period of treatment.

Vitamin B_{12}

The use of vitamin B_{12} as a treatment measure does appear to be of some benefit in MS. This vitamin is required for the formation of myelin and for immune mechanisms, and it has been found to be important in the recovery of the spinal cord from other causes of degeneration. Studies have found that MS patients tend to have significantly lower vitamin B_{12} levels than normal, and sometimes a person with MS will show a clear deficiency. There is some evidence from controlled research studies that injections of vitamin B_{12} can lead to an improvement in MS abnormalities, according to measurements in visual and brainstem auditory evoked potentials; and it has also been found that a massive dose of B_{12} therapy may be useful as an adjunct to immunosuppressive treatment for chronic progressive MS. In practice, therefore, injections of this vitamin are often prescribed for MS patients during relapses.

Diet

Another line of treatment has been diet, covered more fully in Chapter 6. Of particular interest is the evidence from a number of studies that people with MS appear to have a deficiency in the level of polyunsaturated fats in their bodies, especially linoleic acid contained, for example, in sunflower seed oil. Diets have been designed to help in providing a richer intake of polyunsaturated fats while reducing the consumption of saturated fats. A number of studies have demonstrated the value of such diets for MS sufferers, as discussed in Chapter 6. Gluten-free diets (which are essential in the treatment of coeliac disease) have also been tried, but no clear beneficial effects on MS have been demonstrated in clinical trials.

Cannabis

There has been a good deal of media coverage of the possible value of cannabis as a form of treatment in MS, and several sufferers have claimed that smoking marijuana acts as a much more effective relaxant in the reduction of spasms than other medications prescribed for their condition. But there is also evidence that the drug can have negative side effects, such as the impairment of posture and balance, and so far very little clinical evidence has been produced in support of its use in MS. A synthetic cannaboid drug called Nabilone (taken orally) has also been tried in a few individual MS cases, with varying effects. Its main benefit again appears to be a reduction in discomfort from muscle spasm. However, the drug is only obtainable by prescription from hospitals, where its main use is as an anti-emetic for patients undergoing chemotherapy. Properly conducted clinical trials are needed to establish whether cannabis or one of the synthetic cannaboid drugs has a role to play in the treatment of MS.

Hyperbaric oxygen

In the late 1970s considerable interest was aroused in the use of hyperbaric oxygen to treat MS sufferers. Oxygen breathed at increased atmospheric pressure (that is, hyperbaric oxygen) produces a high concentration of oxygen in the body, and this has been shown to be of some benefit, for example, in treating neurological lesions following head injury. It was thought that it might also be of benefit in MS, and by the early 1980s treatment was being provided in centres across the country, using pressure chambers similar to those used by deep-sea divers.

Since there are risks associated with hyperbaric treatment, especially for MS patients who suffer from chronic ear or sinus disease, asthma, chronic bronchitis or emphysema, it was considered important that the treatment should be scientifically evaluated. Various trials were set up in Britain and overseas. At the beginning of 1986 a paper was published reporting the results of one of these trials, funded by the MS Society, and involving two London teaching hospitals.[16] During the trial the experimental group breathed oxygen at twice atmospheric pressure while in a pressurised chamber, whereas the placebo group breathed normal air in the same conditions but at a different time. Each group received twenty treatment sessions over a four-week period. The results were disappointing. No significant improvements were found in the patients who had received the oxygen, although a few had a slightly increased bladder capacity. Both groups of patients experienced unwanted effects from the treatment, minor ear discomfort and fatigue being the commonest. A number of people with MS still pursue treatment with hyperbaric oxygen and claim to feel some benefit from it. But the results from the London trial, and from other trials in the UK and elsewhere, unfortunately do not support its general use in the management of MS.[17]

Other treatments

Several other treatments have been or are currently being investigated as possible treatments for MS. For example, some benefits have been claimed from the use of a synthetic product designed to interfere with the demyelination process. This is co-polymer 1 (or COP-1), which has been shown in trials to reduce frequency of relapses. A UK licence for use of this particular drug is expected soon. Experiments have also been carried out on the effects of stimulating the dorsal area of the spinal cord by electrodes. There was some indication that this form of treatment might improve, at least temporarily, some body functions, including the bladder in the more severely disabled. However, the results overall have been disappointing, and there are also risks of infection associated with the treatment. Some success has been achieved, on the other hand, using neuromuscular stimulation of the muscles of the lower leg. Preliminary results suggest that the use of electrodes placed over the muscles, building up to two half-hour sessions a day, may improve neuromuscular performance, walking ability and endurance in some MS patients with walking difficulties.[18]

Another approach to treatment has been developed on the assumption that immunity can be transferred from one person to another by injecting an extract of white blood cells (leukocytes). Thus MS patients have been given injections of a white blood cell extract (called 'transfer factor') obtained from relatives living with them. Despite the fact that relapses continued to occur in patients treated with the extract, the early findings suggested that this treatment might help to slow down the progression of the disease in patients with mild to moderate disability. Unfortunately, longer-term follow-up research studies have been disappointing, and the benefits have not been maintained. There has also been some suggestion that mercury toxicity from silver dental fillings (amalgam) may have an adverse effect in MS and that there may be benefit in having these fillings removed and replaced by the 'white' non-amalgam type. One or two studies do appear to show a trend whereby patients who have had their amalgam removed have a lower rate of relapse, but this is by no means an established finding.

For the majority of different kinds of symptoms that might trouble MS sufferers, drug treatments are, of course, the same as those given to persons with other health problems. For example, antibiotics are given for urinary infections, and anti-spasmodic drugs such as oxybutynin for minor urinary incontinence; Imodium can be used for bowel frequency or incontinence, while Colofac can relieve pain associated with frequent bowel movements; and counselling, combined with tranquillisers or anti-depressants where necessary, would be offered to people with severe emotional difficulties. As far as pain management is concerned, this again is usually dealt with by the normal approaches to pain relief, and your GP or Consultant will be able to offer advice on suitable medication. In general, MS is not a disorder which inflicts unbearable pain, although the incidence of pain and discomfort is often underestimated. A nagging pain of a toothache kind is not uncommon, muscular spasms produce uncomfortable 'tightening' effects, and other MS episodes can sometimes bring on similar cramp-like pains or an involuntary and painful contraction of the facial muscles on one side that lasts for a few seconds. Also, MS sufferers sometimes have to put up with intense itching, confined to a specific area of skin. Like the facial contraction, this can be triggered by movement (e.g. touching the part of the body involved). Such discomfort often tends to occur quite frequently for a period and then to go into remission.

Looking to the future

The breakthrough in the medical treatment of many common diseases (such as gout and stomach ulcers) tends to result, of course, from the 'brick-by-brick' accumulation of new information over a number of years by scientists in various specialised fields. For multiple sclerosis this pattern of joint research is now in progress. The two major funding bodies in this country are the Multiple Sclerosis Society of Great Britain and Northern Ireland, and the government's Medical Research Council. In addition, there is international co-operation through both scientific journals and conferences, and the International Federation of Multiple Sclerosis Societies. Through these co-operative efforts very considerable progress has been made in the past decade in understanding viral diseases, the immunological processes in the body, and the pathology of the central nervous system – all of which have a direct relevance to multiple sclerosis.

Research in the 1990s has also begun to reveal some enormously exciting possibilities, not least the prospect that within a few years it might be possible to repair damage to the myelin sheath. In the meantime, until the mystery of MS begins to unravel more fully and doctors are able to intervene to arrest, or even reverse, the progress of the disease, physiotherapy remains the cornerstone of treatment –

encouraging people to select suitable forms of exercise to help in maintaining physical fitness. In this way, MS sufferers can help to make the most of the strengths that they possess, and maintain (or improve) their levels of general health. This will ensure that they are in good shape to take full advantage of the treatments which are now beginning to emerge. It is also important to assist the body in fighting the disease by paying close attention to other aspects of general life-style, particularly diet, which have been shown to be of benefit in MS. You can think of diet and exercise as the two 'tigers in your tank' which will help fight off the enemy until rescue is at hand! We shall return to these fighting tigers in Chapter 6.

3
MS and the family

MS sometimes strikes before thoughts of marriage or starting a family have become important. More usually, however, it appears at a time when two people may be contemplating marriage or planning to have a family. For the couple about to get married the burning issue is what effect MS is likely to have on their married life.

MS and marriage

As mentioned in the previous chapter, MS is neither an infectious nor a contagious disease and there is therefore no danger of its transmission from one partner to the other. It is a disease, however, which makes great demands upon sufferers and their close family and friends. Some people find disability of any sort difficult to contend with and may shrink away from the prospect of painful emotional or physical experiences. As noted, MS does not generally inflict unbearable pain, but it does present considerable problems of adjustment in social, financial, sexual and emotional matters. Such adjustments are generally much easier to make in the context of a loving and supportive relationship as, for example, in a good marriage. If the bond between two people is sufficiently strong and based upon values and interests which are not just transitory, then marriage with MS can be a great success despite the difficulties. If the bonds between two individuals are flimsy, however, and based upon little more than physical attraction, the chances of maintaining a steady relationship in the midst of MS are much less good. The decision about whether to marry or not must be an individual decision based upon careful consideration of the circumstances. To write off marriage or living together simply because one partner has this disease would be a very shallow way of looking at the problem, and there are many instances of highly successful and fulfilled marriages or relationships in which one partner has MS.

Coming to terms with the diagnosis

The first problem facing anyone with MS is how to accept the initial diagnosis. This can often be a devastating experience. Sometimes the information is acquired when the person is least ready to accept it (for example, when suffering from a sudden relapse or when in hospital for another apparently unconnected complaint). It would be helpful if some form of counselling support were available within the health service at such times, but constructive advice tends to be very limited. Some GPs are very good and some nurses or social workers can be helpful at such a time of stress. The local branch of the MS Society or the MS Helpline[1] can also be of great assistance; the opportunity to talk with another MS sufferer can be a considerable help.

The first thing to accept, of course, is that it is quite natural to feel depressed and even rather desperate on first hearing about MS. On examining the possible consequences of the disease, however, it usually becomes clear that the picture which is sometimes painted of rapid and drastic deterioration in the condition is less than accurate in most cases.

The very worst thing to do would be to look in an out-of-date medical dictionary at this time! Before you know where you are you will be condemned to a wheelchair as a prelude to becoming permanently bedridden in no time at all. Fortunately, the majority of MS cases are less dramatic! There may be very little disability in the early stages. Difficulty in walking and perhaps some urgency in needing to go to the toilet may be the main problems at such a stage, and in some cases a remission can mean that the person does not even suffer these limitations. People often find it helpful to talk about their anxieties openly to their partner or to an understanding doctor, social worker or MS society member. Many of the worst fears are unfounded and it is important to try to obtain a reliable picture of the sort of problems with which the MS sufferer has to cope. It is also important to realise that the period of adjustment to the initial medical diagnosis of MS will differ in length according to the individual concerned. For most people it seems to take about two years before it is possible to talk easily to relatives and friends about the illness. The feelings of fear, anger and inadequacy which are often very strong at first wear off in time, and it becomes easier and easier to discuss the problems of MS with other people. The illness can then become a challenge to which many people both inside and outside the family will respond most strongly – and don't forget that in many cases the symptoms subside for long periods (sometimes permanently) and that in others they will remain fairly static or even improve. So the story is often less gloomy than it might at first appear.

The role of the partner in MS

There is sometimes an understandable tendency for the partner (or carer) of an MS sufferer to 'mollycoddle the invalid'. In many cases this has the unfortunate effect of reducing the degree of independence of the person with MS, who becomes labelled as a 'patient' incapable of carrying out normal household or occupational activities. This can lower the morale of the person and in certain ways lead to a deterioration in his or her physical condition. In fighting this illness it is extremely important that the MS sufferer should keep as fully involved in the activities formerly engaged in for as long as possible. For example, gardening, cooking or cleaning might take a great deal longer than they used to, but the exercise that such activities provide for mind and muscles is extremely important in the maintenance of physical and mental well-being. Watching the person with MS doing jobs at an excruciatingly slow pace can be most frustrating for the onlooker as well as the individual. Too frequently this leads the onlooker to exclaim 'let me do it' and to take over the task which is consequently accomplished much more swiftly. It is phrases and actions such as these which require curbing on the part of the able-bodied partner. Nothing can dent the morale of an MS sufferer more than the gradual loss of responsibilities. Rather than take over the task it is often more constructive to try to find ways of making that task easier (for example, by using a long-handled trowel for gardening or an electric mixer or food processor instead of a wooden spoon when cooking).

In general it is true, however, that for every disabled person it is helpful if there is someone around who is able-bodied. One of the adjustments which the MS sufferer has to make is to learn to accept help when it is needed. This is often a most difficult adjustment to make. Many people with MS become fiercely independent and sometimes seem to reject offers of help in a startlingly brusque manner. To those who live with MS this might be accepted simply as an assertion of independence; to those unconnected with MS it appears to be rudeness. The person with MS needs to come to terms with the fact that help is sometimes required and to accept it gracefully.

In the situation where partners' roles can often be virtually reversed it is not surprising that tensions will creep into the relationship. Such tensions are perfectly natural. People with MS often tend to feel guilty about the extra burden which is being placed on their partner. On the other hand, the able-bodied partner may sometimes feel annoyed and resentful at having to forgo leisure activities because of family commitments. The husband or wife can sometimes also be over-sensitive to criticism. A husband may feel, for example, that he is doing enough simply to take on some extra household chores without being criticised for doing them in a manner which is at variance with his wife's usual approach. People with MS in these circumstances have to accept that tasks which they have previously performed to their own particular standards will now be performed by their partner in *his* or *her* own way. It is often small points like the way in which clothes are hung out on the line or how the car is cleaned which will present the most irritating points of conflict. Pride has often to be swallowed and critical tongues bitten in order to cope with such tensions. Given understanding and good humour, however, they need not become permanent complications.

MS does not respect privacy in a marriage. One of the things people with MS may have to accept is the necessity of allowing the partner to help with some of the body's basic functions. Difficulty in reaching the toilet on time can be a problem in MS and coupled with the difficulty in physical movement of arms and legs this may make assistance with clothing necessary. Bathing, getting in and out of bed, sometimes eating and drinking – all these may require assistance to a greater or lesser degree. 'And one man in his time plays many parts.' (*As You Like It*, Act II, scene 7.)

Sexual relations between partners need not necessarily be affected by MS. The functioning of the body in this respect may remain perfectly normal, although there may be difficulties in some cases. Occasionally, male sufferers may find impotence occurs. This is not, of course, only a problem for MS sufferers, and it is worth consulting the GP to see if it is something which may be amenable to treatment. And for women with MS some loss of sensation may also sometimes occur. But even if it is not always easy to treat these problems, the possibility of engaging in satisfactory sexual relations is not something to discard. Of course, the giving and receiving of sexual pleasure is not confined to penetrative sexual intercourse alone, and couples can achieve intense enjoyment of sex, including orgasm, through other forms of mutual or self-stimulation of the genital organs. Sexual pleasure can also be derived simply from the warmth of close physical contact with one's partner. A hug and a kiss can give a tremendous feeling of physical and emotional reassurance to both partners; and added mutual pleasure can be achieved by caressing various parts of the body through a gentle stroking with fingers, lips or tongue or indeed any other part of the anatomy! In fact, some couples in which one of the partners has MS have found that their sexual experiences have improved since they have had to experiment with different forms of love-making! There are a number of very useful pamphlets giving advice on sexual matters for disabled people, produced by the MS Society and by SPOD.[2]

One of the main problems in sexual matters is physical discomfort and fatigue. The claim that 'I'm too tired tonight' is something which tends to have rather more justification in MS than might always be the case in other situations! As in other aspects of the relationship, therefore, adjustments have to be made.

A final point on the relationship between partners concerns the fact that many MS sufferers are unable to leave the house on their own. In these circumstances the able-bodied partner often acts as the eyes and ears of the person with MS. It is important to spend time discussing things which are taking place in the local town or village so that the MS sufferer feels involved in the outside world. Visits to places of interest or even a drive around the houses with no particular destination in mind can be like a trip to Buckingham Palace to see the Queen for somebody who is generally housebound. It is important also to try to overcome the embarrassment an able-bodied partner may feel when taking their MS partner to social occasions. MS sufferers have the problem of coming to terms with their own self-image as disabled, and their partners have the parallel problem of adjusting to the disability and to other people's reactions to it. In order to come to terms with this problem it is sometimes necessary to force oneself into accepting invitations despite initial reservations. As time progresses and the circle of understanding acquaintances increases, social activities become easier to cope with. At this stage fatigue is more a problem than embarrassment.

Children and MS

The question about whether or not to have children is one which some people with MS have to face. Medical opinion in general gives no strong guidance either way. Adoption agencies, on the other hand, tend to reject parents with MS on the grounds that they have enough able-bodied applicants to provide their children with adoptive parents. The disease is not directly inherited and the fact that there is a 'familial tendency' in MS (i.e. relatives have a slightly higher risk of developing the disease than non-relatives) is not regarded by most doctors as sufficient grounds for discouraging an MS couple from having children. As far as pregnancy is concerned in a woman with MS, medical advice needs to be sought with respect to each individual case. Occasionally pregnancy may be inadvisable e.g. on grounds of poor general health; on the other hand there are many cases in which pregnancy and childbirth appear to have little or no effect on the course of the disease. Indeed, there is a good deal of evidence to suggest that women with MS actually have fewer relapses during their pregnancies and tend to feel well. Taken together with the small-scale study suggesting that women on HRT also tend to experience an improvement of symptoms these findings lend support to the view that hormonal factors may be implicated in some way in MS. As one woman put it: 'I felt extremely well all the way through my pregnancy . . . The only problem was the extra weight I was carrying. It slowed down my walking to snail's pace!' It is the period following the child's birth which creates the greatest problem for the mother with MS. For a mother in good health this period is very fatiguing; for the mother with MS it becomes even more fatiguing and the family need to rally round at this time to give as much assistance as possible.

The other general consideration the prospective parents have to bear in mind is whether it is right to bring a child into the world into circumstances where the couple may find it difficult to cope with the upbringing of children because of the disability, or where the family may be at risk financially because of a parent's illness. Each case needs to be considered on its own merits. However, any disadvantages to the child's upbringing which may result from the physical frailty of a parent or from financial hardship will be more than offset in the long term by the security and emotional warmth provided by a loving family.

In making a decision about whether or not to have children it is wise to take into account the long-term as well as the short-term future, to make sure that the decision is a joint one and that there are people within the family who would help out in times of difficulty. Family planning also becomes very important in the case of families where one of the members has MS. This is another reason why it is important for sufferers to be told they have MS as soon as the symptoms are well established and a firm diagnosis has been made.

In general the children of MS families seem to develop healthily and happily. There are, however, certain aspects of growing up which such children might miss out on. For example, it is not as easy for a parent with MS to take the children out or to visit school functions as it is for an able-bodied parent. Children have to learn to be independent at an early age and this can often be a great aid to the development of maturity. It can also sometimes lead to a feeling that they are being imposed upon. The danger of placing too much responsibility on the children is something of which MS parents (perhaps mothers in particular) are often acutely aware. The parents may also sometimes feel rather guilty that they are not able to do everything they would like for their children because of the limitations imposed by the disability.

There is, however, a very *positive* side to bringing up children in a family where one parent has MS. Living with disability seems to give children a sensitivity to the needs of other people which is less easily acquired in able-bodied families. If children have known their parents as MS sufferers from their early childhood then it is likely that they will accept the disability and its consequences without too much frustration or embarrassment.

Children can often be disconcertingly frank. Whereas adults will refrain from remarking upon abnormalities of physique or gait for fear of embarrassing, the inquisitive child will simply ask in a straightforward way 'Why do you walk like that?' or 'Why have you got a stick?' Such curiosity is best answered by straightforward explanations: 'I've got a funny leg'; 'My legs won't work properly'. As the children get older more precise information about MS can be discussed, and children show a good understanding of the problems involved and will often spend time thinking how to cope with them. For example, one little boy friendly with a family in which the mother has MS always looked to see if the places he visited on school and family outings were accessible for a wheelchair. The daughter of an MS mother exclaimed: 'When I grow up I'm going to buy a house without any steps so that mummy will be able to come and visit me.' Wheelchairs are constant sources of interest to children. Unlike many adults who seem to shun people in wheelchairs out of embarrassment, children seem drawn towards them out of wonder and curiosity at this interesting form of transport.

Some children of MS parents may show an excessive degree of anxiety about their parent's condition, and anger at the 'loss' of the parent they used to have (the Dad who used to run around and play football with them or the Mum who always used to take them to school, now both events of the past). Others may worry about whether they will get the disease themselves, despite being reassured that MS is not passed on directly from parent to child and that it cannot be 'caught'. It's important to realise that such feelings of anxiety, frustration and anger are quite natural, and it is helpful for children to be able to express their worries openly. Just as the parents have to find ways of coming to terms with the impact of MS on their lives, so the children need time to adjust to *their* new situation. (The MS Society has produced a useful booklet on MS, specifically written for children, called *Has your Mum or Dad got MS?* This is available from the MS Society – address in Chapter 8).

In cases where adjustment proves particularly difficult, the GP may consider arranging for some form of family counselling, but over a period of time most children seem to accept the changed situation in a fairly well balanced way. They will have their periods of anxiety about what would happen if there was a fire, whether mummy will have to go into hospital, what happens if daddy dies – but these are not greatly different from the fears and worries of children in ordinary households. The drawbacks which children suffer from having a parent who is more housebound than most other parents are counterbalanced by advantages such as the likelihood that this parent will usually be at home when the child comes home from school! In general the development of independence, responsibility and sensitivity to the needs of others seem great bonuses to set against the minor frustrations.

The role of relatives and friends

The parents of MS sufferers often seem to feel as much of a shock as the patients themselves at the time of the initial diagnosis. It is also the experience of MS sufferers that parents are often among the most difficult with whom to discuss the illness because of their emotional involvement. They sometimes seem not to want to talk about the disease and pretend that it is not there. Another reaction is to want to take the person back in to the parental home so that they can look after them 'properly'. This overprotective urge is something which parents need to guard against. Although the task of looking after a daughter or son with MS may fulfil a parental need it can also reduce the independence of the individual MS sufferer. For the parent, pushing their daughter or son around in a wheelchair may seem a helpful and unselfish gesture, but to the person in the wheelchair it may seem too closely related to childhood experiences to be seen in this way. The person with MS will usually appreciate the 'unfussy' approach much more than the 'cottonwool treatment', even though this may seem slightly harsh to the parents. This is how one MS sufferer puts it:

> The most important attitude of all . . . in dealing with those of us who are handicapped, is that which treats us as far as possible as if we enjoyed normal health . . . It is certainly my experience that we who are handicapped are happier and healthier if, up to a point, we are 'treated rough', and not only encouraged but *expected* to do things for ourselves, without any fuss or comment being made about what we do.

Relatives generally can be a tremendous source of support to the family with MS if they try to understand the particular problems of MS, such as fatigue. They can often provide a very effective back-up service to the immediate family, stepping in as 'babysitters' or 'food suppliers' or 'transporters' at times of difficulty. Close friends can also be tremendously helpful. It's not the person who goes on her 'do-gooding' visit with a bunch of flowers who is of most value to the MS sufferer, but the friend who says 'I'm just going shopping – is there anything I can get you?' The flower person fatigues, the shopper prevents fatigue. The real friend is one who is willing to come in and mop up the dog's puddle because the person with MS can't get down to do this. It is helpful also for friends to remember that sitting chatting over a cup of tea for a couple of hours can be extremely tiring for some people with MS. Another important point is that the ordinary colds and 'flus which most people take in their stride may be more of a problem for the person with MS. A bout of 'flu can be very debilitating for an MS sufferer and it is, therefore, important that people should not bring such germs into the household where someone has MS.

It is quite common for people to find that they lose one or two friends after MS has been diagnosed. Some probably are unable to face up to any discussion of illness and keep away out of fear and embarrassment. Other friends seem to be insufficiently aware of the nature of the disease. The main problem of MS, according to one sufferer, is 'trying to explain to other people why I can't do the things I used to'!

In some circumstances, of course, the MS sufferer may prefer to live alone and to be independent of the family. In such situations it may be possible to arrange a means-tested 'community care package' from the Social Services. The Disablement Income Group (DIG) has also produced a useful booklet which discusses how to recruit and employ a personal care worker.[3] For most MS sufferers, however, the family is likely to remain the major source of help and support; and although MS clearly has very considerable effects on family life it is important to stress that there are very many families coping successfully with the problems. Indeed, some families have come closer together as a consequence of them.

4
Coping and hoping (1): In the home

In MS one has to cope with the immediate consequences of the disease while at the same time keeping alive the hope that research will come up with the cause and some further pointers to treatment. It is therefore very much a position of coping and hoping. In this chapter we shall look at ways of coping in the home, and in Chapter 5 at the issues with which the person with MS has to cope when 'out and about'.

General problems

As far as coping is concerned, this depends very much upon the nature of the symptoms in each particular case. It also depends upon the home circumstances and the stage of the illness. For example, the requirements for coping with someone in a wheelchair are rather different from those in which the person is able to walk short distances. The symptoms are many and varied, but there are one or two features which seem common to most people with MS – fatigue, poor balance and difficulty in walking, for example, are basic problems. MS sufferers sometimes have difficulty in locating their limbs in relation to the rest of their body; pins and needles and heaviness of the limbs are also common. These symptoms lead to many instances of dropped crockery and headlong falls after tripping over carpets or pavements. Fingers sometimes lack sensation and may become progressively weaker in grasping objects and poorer in close coordination. This can lead to difficulty in dressing, performing ordinary household tasks such as cutting bread, sewing, hairwashing. These sorts of problems do not, of course, all occur at the same time, and some people with MS may only ever experience a very small range of symptoms; the list in this chapter is not a description of the inevitable! MS is a very individual disease affecting people in all sorts of different ways, and the fact that certain symptoms *can* appear doesn't mean that they *will* appear in each case. It is also important to remember that some of the symptoms which an MS sufferer may be experiencing now may well disappear later. In other words, people with MS can, and often do get better as well as worse:

Twenty years ago I was stuck in a wheelchair most of the time. But

> I've gradually improved over the last ten years and I now walk about with just a stick. I'm so much better I'm thinking of starting to drive again!

Some of the other problems which can appear in MS relate to extremes of temperature. For example, circulation is often poor and this can lead to excessively cold or excessively hot feet and hands and some swelling of the limbs. MS sufferers can also be adversely affected by hot sun. Sometimes vision may be impaired (by temporary bouts of double vision) and this can affect leisure pursuits such as reading or watching television. People with MS can also have problems with cramps, 'floppy' limbs or stiffness of the muscles. Stiffness, or excessive muscular tone, is a very common problem which can affect mobility in many ways. For example, in the morning some MS sufferers find that their legs are as stiff as planks at first, and before they can get up from bed they will need assistance in bending their legs. Physical discomfort can also affect sleeping at night. Frequency and urgency in going to the toilet are also common and very difficult problems, as is the general overriding problem of fatigue.

Another problem, especially in the early stages of MS, is that many of the symptoms, such as fatigue and weakness in bladder control, are invisible to other people.

> The presence of these invisible symptoms may cause anxiety, and the patient may not know whether to perceive himself as 'disabled' or 'fit'. He may alternate between the two roles depending on domestic and work circumstances. Sometimes he fails to make allowances for the disease . . . by working too hard or by engaging in stressful activities to prove that he is 'normal'. He may think that if he mentions his tiredness or subjective symptoms he will be regarded as a hypochondriac or as a malingerer.[1]

This description may be representative of the state of mind of some MS sufferers early on in the course of the disease. But over a period of time people with MS, their families, workmates and friends gradually come to terms with the symptoms, both visible and invisible, and many of the conflicts tend to resolve themselves.

With such a range of symptoms, however, it is difficult to give general guidance about coping strategies, and this chapter and the next will take different aspects of everyday life in turn and try to offer certain hints which might be of help to people with MS. There are, however, one or two general comments which might be of help. Perhaps the most important practical step that can be taken is to try to make the physical side of life as convenient as possible. Since lack of mobility and a tendency to become overtired are central features in the illness it is common sense to try to equip the home with as many labour-saving devices as possible. Another general point is the need to avoid over-tiredness. This means planning one's day well in advance and as carefully as possible, so that periods of work can be interspersed with periods of rest throughout the day. If MS is regarded as a challenge and tackled positively and constructively it is usually possible to find ways of coping with even the most difficult problems.

Stress and MS

We have seen that MS can cause stress between sufferers and their partner or family. There may be an undercurrent of hidden tension arising from issues which have not been openly discussed, revealing itself, for example, in petty arguments, persistent nagging and 'critical sniping'. If such a destructive atmosphere is allowed to rumble on it can rapidly lead to soured personal relationships. Problems must be discussed as openly as possible in order to avoid a build-up of suppressed anger and resentment destructive both to the person feeling these emotions and those against whom they are directed.

There does not appear to be any consistent finding that stressful events affect people with MS more strongly than other people. However, the fact that stress will tend to exacerbate the feelings of fatigue in MS provides a warning that leading too stressful a life may sometimes worsen the condition. There does sometimes appear to be a direct link between a traumatic event such as a twisted ankle, a bad fall, an emotionally stressful time or a viral infection, and the onset (or exacerbation) of MS symptoms. But when this has been examined in large-scale studies the evidence does not support any clear causal link,[2] although there is some indication that viral infections and neurosurgery may occasionally lead to an increase in exacerbation rates. With most traumatic events, however, it seems likely that it is MS symptoms such as weakness in a limb or general fatigue which have led to the event rather than the other way round.

Physical health

Since the physical health of MS sufferers is already impaired by the disease it is crucial to try to keep the general level of health as high as possible. In this respect it is helpful to lead a life with as few extra stresses as possible and with as much activity as is compatible with the avoidance of over fatigue. Detailed suggestions on keeping fit and well, and a suitable diet, are given in Chapter 6.

Working from home

General questions about employment for people with MS are discussed in the next chapter. It is worth mentioning at this point, however, that there are a number of possibilities for home-based employment which are worth exploring for those people who have found it difficult to meet the demands of a job in the workplace. For some people, work involving making or receiving telephone calls, or handling mail order material, have proved manageable tasks; and for a teacher who took early retirement, acting as a home tutor for students and marking exam papers provided interesting employment which could be pursued from home. For a number of people, voluntary work has been found to be a rewarding way of keeping up active involvement in their local community. Some have offered their services to their local Citizens' Advice Bureau. Others have become involved with various charities, such as the local branch of the MS Society, where they have been able to help with secretarial duties, telephone counselling, transport/events organising, all of which can be carried out from home. Even more elaborate options are open for some people, and one MS sufferer even ran a business from his home with the aid of a Possum machine.

Housework

The main guideline here is to invest in labour-saving devices. For people with MS, domestic appliances such as freezers, automatic washing machines and tumble driers take on the mantle of household necessities. Unfortunately, they are also expensive necessities which some people with MS may find it hard to afford. This is where some of the local charities, including the MS Society, can sometimes help. The local authority Social Services may also be able to assist with some home conversions or gadgets. One very difficult problem for MS sufferers, for example, is the retrieval of objects from the floor. If they try to bend down to pick them up they inevitably land up on the floor themselves and are unable then to haul themselves back into the chair! One gadget which Community Nurses can supply is a pick-up stick which has a long handle and acts like pincers. They can also supply certain walking aids to provide stability for the MS sufferer. Where available the Community Occupational Therapist will be able to give advice on this.

Making beds is another problem for people with MS. They are often unable to bend down to the level of the bed without toppling over and if one hand is weak then tucking in bedclothes becomes an impossibility. One answer here is to invest in continental quilts. Hanging out clothes on the washing line is another problem for some people with MS. A tumble drier will remove the necessity for this activity if finances and space permit. A helpful neighbour is another possibility. For someone who can just manage to reach the washing line it might be easier to put the clothes pegs on the clothes before approaching the line. Putting the clothes on a trolley and wheeling this to the clothes line is also something which some people have found helpful. Indeed, trollies, provided they are reasonably sturdy and stable, are transports of magnificent worth for anyone suffering from MS. They provide a ready-built walking frame, a conveyor of food and drink, and a most effective extension of the hands and arms when carrying clothes, plants, books from one part of the house to another. It is also possible to obtain wheeled walking frames with a basket attached. These aids are discussed in the next chapter in the section on mobility.

When it comes to ironing the answer is to sit down at the ironing board – a procedure which seems to leave many stand-up traditionalists aghast! The other solution to ironing is to buy clothes which in general are of the 'non-iron' variety – polycotton sheets, drip-dry shirts and so on. If you have the opportunity to decide where electric sockets are placed then it is helpful to raise these a couple of feet or so off the ground so that they are more accessible to a disabled person. For example, if the person is in a wheelchair then he or she would still be able to plug in a vacuum cleaner and push it in front of the wheelchair.

Another aid to housework is the home help, and a great many people with MS have found the local authority service helpful in this respect. One MS sufferer describes her home help as 'an absolute necessity and ministering angel'. The home help can provide a regular social contact as well as a housework, shopping and cooking aid.

Cooking

The weakness in the hands of many MS sufferers can cause problems

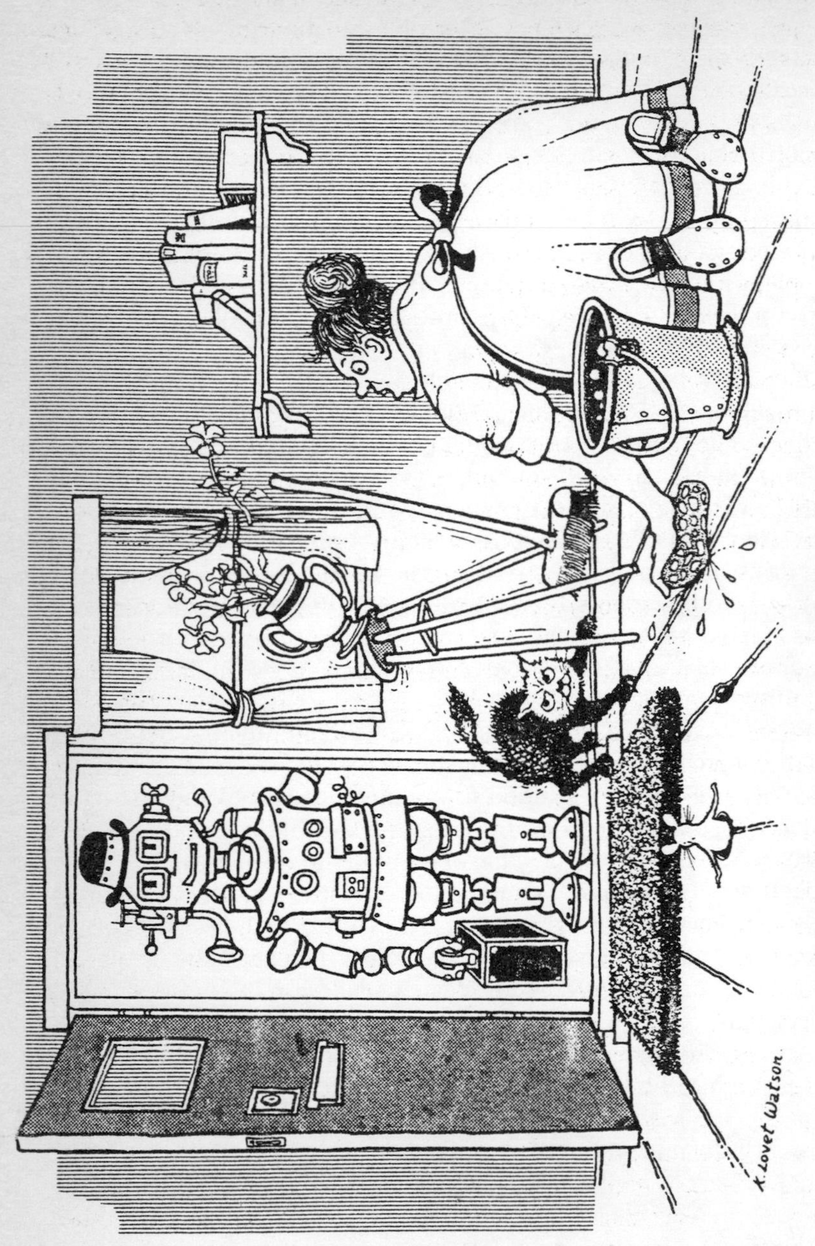

The main guideline here is to invest in labour-saving devices.

with carrying pans and mixing ingredients, while the problems of fatigue can cause difficulties in preparing regular meals. Everything takes three or four times as long in MS as in an able-bodied context, and this also adds to the problems of fatigue. Thus the use of electrical gadgets is clearly of great assistance in the kitchen (and if finance is a problem don't forget that you can ask for help from organisations such as your local MS branch). The difficult-to-operate tin-opener can be replaced by an electric tin-opener, the wooden spoon and bowl can be replaced by an electric mixer or food processor, the fridge can be supplemented by a freezer, the oven by a microwave. For working on kitchen surfaces it is often helpful to sit on a high stool since standing at the sink or kitchen table can soon result in exhaustion. For MS sufferers with visual impairments it is possible to obtain key pads with 'dimples' for microwaves or other appliances so that the operating buttons can be correctly identified. Similarly, colour coding can be used where appropriate for kitchen items and 'talking scales' are invaluable.

If finances can allow the purchase of a freezer then it is possible to cut down one's work fairly dramatically by preparing several meals at the same time and freezing them. For example, if a casserole or bolognese is being prepared then enough can be cooked for three or four meals to be frozen. The effort involved in preparing this amount is very little more than that involved in preparing for one meal, yet the result will be the production of two or three extra meals for future occasions. The same will apply to cake mixtures and many other foods. Even sandwiches can be frozen in bulk for use at a later date. In this way special occasions such as Christmas and birthdays can be planned well in advance and much of the last minute work and effort can be removed.

Peeling vegetables is something people with MS may find difficult. One solution is to resort to baked potatoes rather than peeled and to sample the wide variety of frozen or tinned vegetables on the market. Packs of low fat oven-baked or frozen chips can also save a great deal of effort. The danger with fat-fried chips is that a pan full of hot fat can be a dangerous hazard in the kitchen. One person with MS fell and struck her head whilst frying chips and lay concussed with a pan of sizzling fat just above her head. She remained there until her husband came home at lunchtime. The moral of this tale seems to be – don't fry chips unless accompanied, or get a member of the family to bring them home from the fish and chip shop! One or two kitchen tips are to cook the vegetables in a chip basket placed in a saucepan of water or use a strainer spoon to take the vegetables from the pan instead of trying to tip out the water first; to put a mixing bowl on a rubber sticking mat or in the sink when mixing; to buy tins of ready-made custard, or make it in the microwave or use the 'porridge method' by mixing the powder with the milk in the pan and heating them up together (instead of mixing the custard in a jug and then pouring on the hot milk). A final hint on cooking from a woman with MS: 'the milkman is quite good in the kitchen . . . he opens tins . . . he gets things out of the deep freeze . . . he zips me up the back'!

Living accommodation

Few people are given the opportunity to design their own homes and fewer still have the opportunity to do so with the knowledge that MS has arrived or is lurking nearby. Most people, therefore, have to make do with the accommodation they have and with various modifications to it. The local authority Social Services Department may well be able to help with these modifications. Detailed information about such local authority assistance is given in Chapter 8, together with other information relevant to living accommodation and the disabled (for example, the availability of housing benefit). It is always necessary, of course, to ascertain the exact nature of the assistance available from your own local authority, since practices tend to vary in different localities. If it is possible to influence decisions about the type of living accommodation to be obtained, however, then there are certain points which it would be helpful to bear in mind. Since difficulty in walking is one of the main problems of MS then facilities downstairs and on the level are a priority. At some point the majority of MS sufferers find stairs difficult to negotiate. If the bedroom is upstairs and the only toilet is upstairs then two of the most important rooms in the house are virtually inaccessible. Chairlifts or lifts designed to provide a direct link between the living room and bedroom accommodation are now being supplied with the aid of some local authorities and these can ease the problems. Similarly, it may be possible to build in a downstairs toilet by converting a stair cupboard or building a porch extension which incorporates a cloakroom and toilet. Local authorities are often willing to advise and assist with such conversions for the disabled. If there is a choice about whether to have a shower installed as a washing facility then advantage should be taken of this since the use of a bath can become increasingly difficult for MS sufferers.

Frequently, a bungalow offers an ideal solution, particularly when it comes to wheelchairs. Wheelchair use also requires a reasonable width in door space, although nowadays with 'slim-line' chairs a

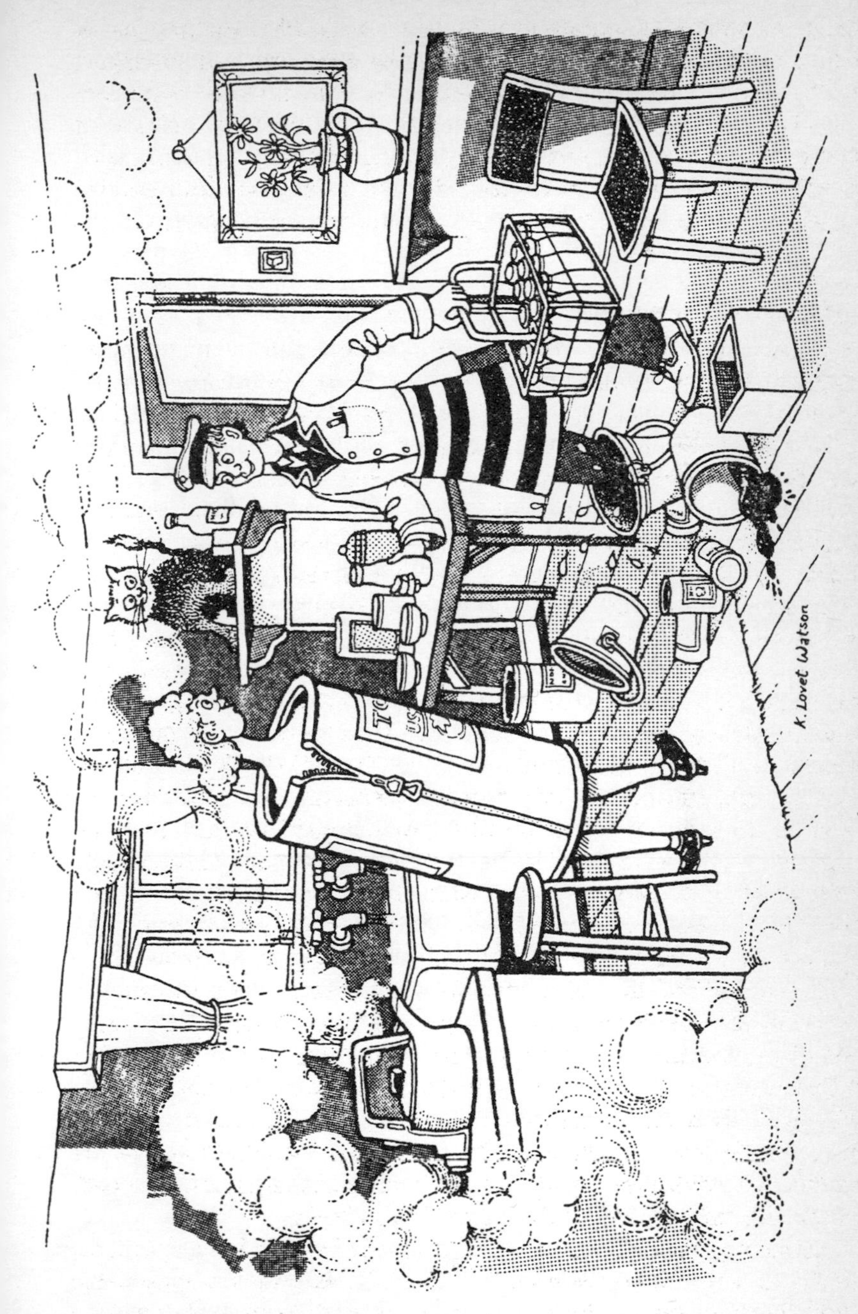

. . . he zips me up the back!

normal door width can be sufficient. Entrance into the house and garage needs to be as level as possible, and even if not required for wheelchair use level or ramped entrances are generally most convenient. Steps are the constant nightmare of people with MS as with other physically handicapped people and the elderly. Slippery floors and rugs are also a danger to the MS sufferer and these are to be avoided.

Kitchen design is something which could be vastly improved in many instances to the benefit of the disabled (and able-bodied) person. Since heavy pans cannot be handled easily it is important that the person with MS should be able to slide the pans from one part of the kitchen to another along a working surface. A useful arrangement is one planned in the following sequence: cooker – surface – sink – surface – fridge. Many people have found split level ovens helpful and also those in which the oven door flap comes down so that it is possible to rest casserole dishes on it.

The phone is also essential. This provides a contact with the outside world and a reassurance of help in times of distress. One problem about the telephone is that the person with MS is often unable to reach the telephone before the caller has rung off. When walking is very impaired this can be a most frustrating experience. The use of a 'cordless' portable telephone is one answer. Another is the careful placement of telephones. For example, a telephone might be placed in the kitchen with a long extension cable so that the telephone can be transported from the kitchen to the lounge by using a trolley. It is possible also to provide extra sockets in other rooms such as the bedroom so the telephone can be moved. It is still worth reminding friends of MS sufferers that they need to keep on ringing to allow the person to reach the phone. The emergency use of the phone can be reduced in effectiveness, of course, if the person trips before reaching the phone. In such circumstances it is useful if the children are well drilled in the '999' call procedure. It has also been found helpful to wear a whistle round the neck so that the attention of a neighbour can be attracted in a way other than by using the phone. More sophisticated electronic devices such as the Peace of Mind or AID-call systems[3] may be offered to disabled people by some Local Authorities. Other systems, such as those produced by Possum and Steeper, may also sometimes be available.[4] One local MS Society member describes her experiences with one such system:

> It was the Occupational Therapist who suggested it in the first place. She thought I'd find a remote control system helpful because I can't

move around easily and I'm always in danger of falling over. The Social Services Department fixed me up with one and I can now switch the lights on and off, operate the television and telephone, and answer the door – all without moving from my chair!

Toilet/washing/dressing

Since problems of frequency and urgency in going to the toilet are prominent in MS, coping with these symptoms is perhaps one of the most important topics to be discussed. One useful rule of thumb is to make sure you empty the bladder fully every few hours. This won't necessarily prevent more frequent visits but it will help to keep down the risk of unexpected leaks! It will also help to keep under control the number of trips which become desperately urgent. As already mentioned, the feeling of urgency is common in MS, exacerbated by the physical difficulty of reaching the toilet quickly. It is crucial, therefore, to make sure that the toilet is readily accessible, and a downstairs loo is clearly a 'must' in most MS homes. Placing a toilet at the top of a steep flight of stairs is like some form of medieval torture to the person with MS! To ascend the stairs at all presents a task of great difficulty; to ascend the stairs with urgency turns the task into a nightmare. As a stopgap measure, portable loos such as those used by campers and caravanners can be very useful (as can pads tucked in the pants). Many MS sufferers have found, for example, that it is helpful to keep a portable toilet by the side of the bed for the first visit of the day. Stiffness in the limbs in the morning can often make even a short walk across the landing very difficult to complete comfortably at that time of the day. Similarly, a portable loo can be a boon in a house where it has not proved possible to incorporate a downstairs toilet.

Urgency or retention can occur, of course, in relation to both bladder and bowels. It is equally important, therefore, to maintain regularity in bowel movements according to the person's own pattern of regularity. With some people this may be once daily; with others more or less frequently. Constipation should be avoided if possible since in MS this often seems to have the effect of weakening bladder control. The attempt to maintain regularity is also important even when the symptoms in MS are at the opposite extreme – hesitancy, retention or difficulty in going to the toilet. There are a number of drugs available for assisting these problems and the GP should be able to advise on these. Occasionally the procedure of self-catheterization is recommended, and some people have found this a very effective solution to their bladder problems. If this is suggested then the technique will be taught to the MS sufferer by the Community Nurse or Continence Adviser, who can also offer helpful suggestions on any of the problems discussed so far in this section.

Washing and bathing in MS can present problems. It is the claim of many MS sufferers that 'I haven't washed my feet for years'! Where the mobility of legs and arms is impaired it can often be almost impossible to reach the feet with the hands. Sometimes by sitting in a chair a person will be able to wash certain parts of the body more easily but even this approach may not always help. Similarly, baths become out of the question for some people, although the Community Nurse may be able to arrange for a 'bathing visit'. Many MS sufferers, however, while finding it possible to lower themselves into the bath find that climbing out afterwards (even with help) proves impossible. There are many stories about MS sufferers taking a bath on their own, letting the water out and then being unable to climb out of the bath without assistance. The window cleaner might well oblige if he or she were in the vicinity, but one cannot always rely on such services! The use of a bath seat (available from the Community Nurse) is sometimes beneficial and 'grab handles' placed on the wall above the bath can be most helpful. Such handles can also be of assistance in other parts of the house (for example, toilet). Some people with MS find that they are able to use a bidet, which can also be useful in washing feet. A home visit from the Community Occupational Therapist can help the MS sufferer to decide upon and acquire the most relevant bathroom and kitchen aids. A range of aids can also be purchased privately from chemists such as Boots, and charitable organisations will sometimes help with expensive items (see Chapter 8).

Perhaps the most valuable piece of washing equipment, however, as mentioned earlier, is the shower. For most people with MS a shower offers the easiest method of all-over washing. For those people who find it difficult to stand under a shower it is possible to incorporate a shower seat. The shower will enable both feet and hair to be washed. Since reaching the feet can still present a problem the long handled brushes or sponges which are available in the shops can be most useful. Similarly, the problem of the 'disappearing soap' can be overcome by using 'soap on a rope'. This again is available in shops and has a loop of rope with a piece of soap on the end so that the rope can hang around the neck and soap is then readily available when required. (Some MS sufferers have found the method of hanging equipment round their necks very helpful in other respects – biros, glasses, bags in which they

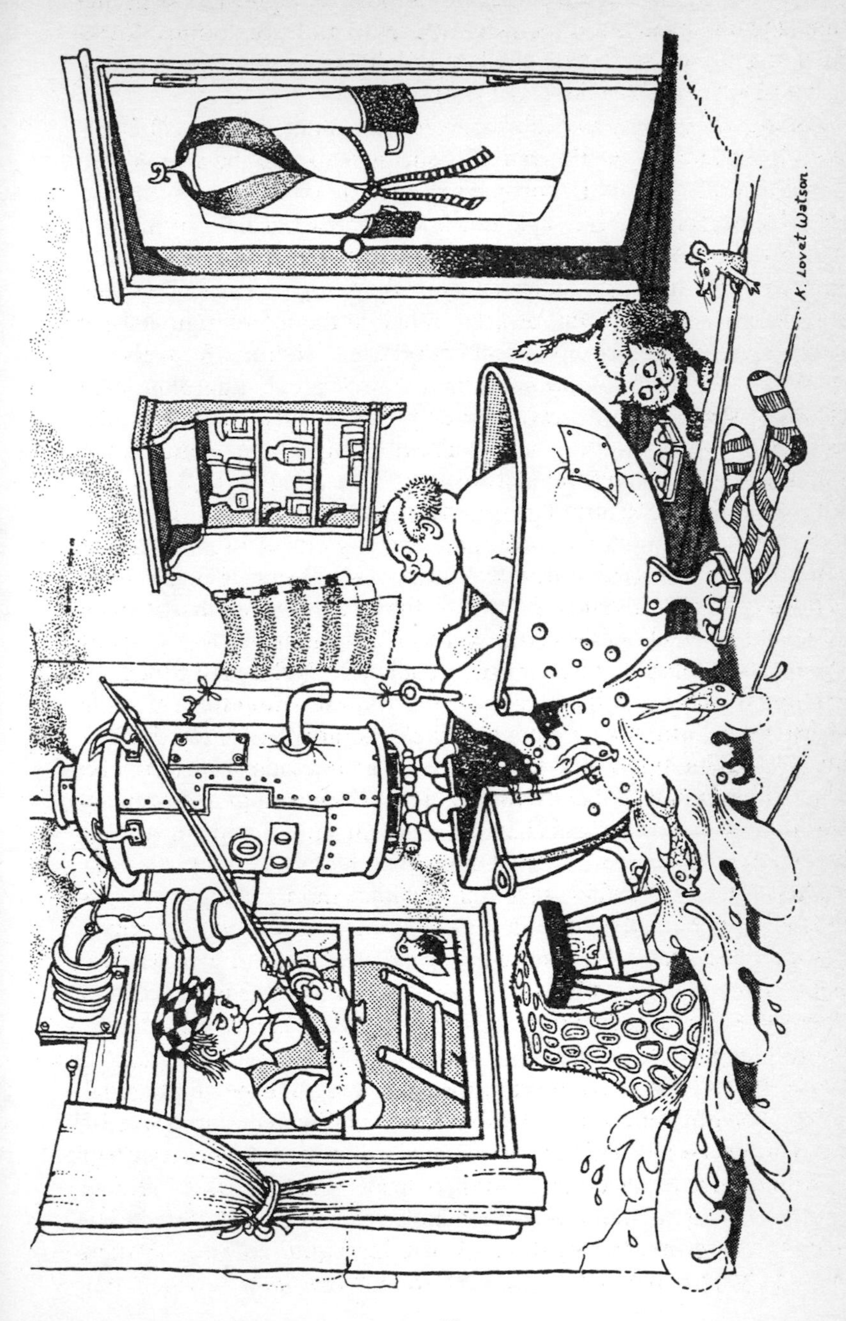

The window cleaner might well oblige . . .

can carry objects from one room to another.) The problem of drying oneself can be helped by using a towelling robe, and some people use a hair drier or fan heater to dry their feet (but not in the bathroom, of course, where it would be electrically unsafe)!

Although the shower might help in washing hair it doesn't necessarily solve the problem of dealing with the hair at the drying and styling stages. For some MS sufferers raising the arms above shoulder level is very tiring and, especially for women, this can create considerable problems in setting their own hair. The assistance of a relative or friend in this exercise is often much appreciated. This can be a welcome social as well as functional occasion. A regular hair shampoo and set in the company of a good friend can be a marvellous tonic. Assistance from family or friends is also valuable in relation to other tasks which MS sufferers may find difficult, such as finger- and toe-nail cutting and shaving. For the housebound, the Community Nurse can arrange visits from a chiropodist.

All the problems of physical immobility which apply to washing also apply to dressing. What takes five minutes for most people will take an hour for someone with MS. Putting on socks or tights can be a major operation. Some people find it useful to dress one half of the body at a time so that one sock or one leg of tights, one leg of the pants and trousers and one shoe would be pulled on first and then the other side. Getting clothes on over the head is often a problem and, therefore, front-opening garments are a help. For women, fastening a bra strap can present an awkward problem, and some people seem to find that the most effective solution is to do the strap up in front and then twist the bra round. Clothes without too many buttons or fasteners are obviously important for people with MS. Velcro can replace zips and is much easier to manage. Trousers with elasticated tops are both easy to get on and to pull down when reaching the toilet. Slip-on shoes or shoes with straps are easier to get on and off than shoes with laces; or elastic shoe laces may be used. As far as nightwear is concerned some people find nightdresses or pyjamas with a slippery texture allow them to turn over in bed more easily.

In this chapter we have considered a whole range of practical suggestions for making it easier to cope with MS in the home. Some of these ideas will also be of help when the person with MS is 'out and about', but there are also a number of respects in which the problems of coping outside the home need to be looked at separately. These will be examined in the next chapter.

5

Coping and hoping (2): Out and about

In general, people with MS try to cope with a normal pattern of life, with minor adjustments here and there, for as long as possible and aim to keep sufficiently fit to be able to take advantage of the hoped-for treatments which are, at last, beginning to emerge. This means that outdoor activities are at least as important as indoor ones, and, in order to cope with these, advice is often required on the best way of dealing with mobility problems.

Mobility

Advice about mobility depends a great deal upon the type of symptoms and their severity, and the Department of Transport have produced an informative book (*Door to door: a guide to transport for disabled people*) which covers all aspects of mobility from aids and benefits to air and sea travel. This book is published by HMSO and available from bookshops or libraries.

For many MS sufferers all that is required is some assistance with balance, and a walking stick will frequently suffice. A child's push-chair can also be of considerable assistance in the early days of MS since this gives a valuable stability in walking. Similarly, shopping trollies, providing they are well oiled and not too full, can help with walking. Another walking aid is the 'walk about',[1] which consists of a frame on wheels to which a shopping basket can be attached; a Uniscan 'A' frame walking aid with a resting seat is also a useful aid.[2]

People with MS can often drive a car either normally or with adapted controls. The Disability Living Allowance is available for MS sufferers and this can be used to help in the purchase of cars (a special Motability scheme is also available for this purpose) or for the payment of taxi fares or to help with transport costs in general (see Chapter 8). Associations such as the Disabled Drivers' Association can help to keep people up to date with the variety of car conversions available. The most common are hand controls. It is also possible, however, to provide such facilities as left-foot accelerator pedals on automatic cars to aid someone with a right-sided weakness. The Mobility Centre, Banstead, and the Mobility Information Service, National Mobility Centre will offer help and advice on choosing an appropriate car or adaptation and are equipped to provide individual assessments. (See Chapter 8.)

If someone with MS is able to drive then tasks such as going to work, shopping and collecting children from school become much easier. Local authorities supply special parking discs to help disabled drivers in parking for longer periods than able-bodied drivers and for stopping at points close to their destination (for example, outside or at the rear entrance of a food store). One of the difficulties, however, which confronts MS sufferers is that the physical effort of reaching a shopping centre can so reduce the store of energy that the shopping itself frequently needs to be greatly curtailed. Parking near to the shop becomes in these circumstances absolutely essential. It is essential also from the point of view of loading shopping into the car. Carrying heavy bags is often an impossibility and assistance may be required for loading the car. Fortunately, many shops are sympathetic to the needs of disabled people in this respect.

A number of towns and cities have also now begun to provide *Shopmobility* schemes for disabled people, and these can be a 'god-send'. They usually operate in a central position in the shopping precinct, sometimes within a multi-storied car park or with disabled parking close by. The schemes allow people with walking difficulties to *borrow* a wheelchair, either self-propelled or powered, for a few hours so that they can visit the town centre without the necessity of bringing their own wheelchair with them. This avoids the need to lift wheelchairs in and out of cars and gives people who may not possess a powered chair the opportunity of using one for shopping expeditions or town centre visits. The freedom this service offers to MS sufferers who use wheelchairs, and their 'pushers', is enormous. It helps to avoid the back strain involved in lifting and pushing wheelchairs and gives the person with walking difficulties a new pair of independent 'legs-on-wheels'.

> I felt 'free as air' when I first went off in the electric wheelchair. I didn't need anyone to push me and I whizzed around the town on my own and went to places I'd never managed to get to before. I even bought my husband a birthday present on my own, without having to arrange a secret mission into town with a friend!

Travelling by bus or train is something which presents difficulties for MS sufferers since both require considerable agility on entering and leaving the vehicle. Rail and coach operators, however, do make special provision for the disabled where possible, and the Disability Discrimination Act (1995) has introduced statutory regulations intended to improve access for disabled people to public transport. One of the hazards of MS is that people may appear perfectly healthy, hence keen bus drivers sometimes shut the doors or move off before they have appreciated the degree of the passenger's disability. The use of a car is therefore likely to be more appropriate for MS sufferers, whether their own car or that of a relative or friend. Many people have found by experience that what appears at first sight to be a very comfortable car may be rather awkward when it comes to ease of access for someone who is physically handicapped. There is no substitute for trying out particular car models for yourself if you are thinking of buying one, but there are one or two general points which might be of help. Most people find it helpful to enter a car by backing in! The person sits on the seat and then brings his or her legs in afterwards. In order to do this comfortably the door needs to open widely and to remain open. Grab handles on the inside can also be helpful to the disabled. The boot should be sufficiently large to take a wheelchair. Estate models or hatch-backs are clearly valuable from this point of view, but most cars are able to accommodate a folding wheelchair.

If the stage comes when someone with MS needs to resort to a wheelchair then a new set of considerations arise. Most people with MS would advise that one should 'keep out of a wheelchair as long as possible'. At some point, however, a wheelchair often becomes a necessity in order to maintain an adequate degree of mobility. The use of a wheelchair for part of the day can also serve to conserve energy for other periods when some standing or walking is necessary. To resort to a wheelchair in such circumstances is far from an admission of defeat. It is a sound and well-proven strategy by which to combat fatigue and conserve energy. Transition to wheelchair-use, however, is psychologically often quite difficult. In a wheelchair which requires to be pushed the person immediately becomes dependent upon the pusher and a certain degree of autonomy has to be surrendered. There is also a tendency on the part of other people to treat the person in the wheelchair as if he or she is mentally as well as physically disabled. The 'Does he take sugar?' phenomenon is very common. Well-meaning people tend to ignore people in wheelchairs as individuals and talk over their heads to their companions. Nothing can be more infuriating and frustrating to the wheelchair-bound person. It is important also to realise that the wheelchair user's view of the outside world remains basically the same as that of the able-bodied except that it is a view from a seated position. Disabled people don't tend, therefore, at first to see the image of themselves as wheelchair-bound unless faced by a mirror or photograph, and this image is one to which they will need time to adjust. Similarly, people who are wheelchair-bound during their waking hours tend in their dreams to be walking, running or flying – but rarely in a wheelchair!

There are also a number of drawbacks and limitations concerning wheelchair design. One MS sufferer sums it up like this:

> If one accepts the premise that a wheelchair is a form of transport, which it is, then one can only stress how very limited is the choice and variety. While there are Boat Shows and Motor Shows that fill Earls Court exhibition hall, the variety of wheelchairs available would fill my sitting room. Babies also are far better catered for than the disabled; for them, imagination and innovation seem to have completely dried up. The baby, for instance, has a hood and a pram cover; the infirm have no protection against the elements whatsoever. The baby faces the pusher; the adult has his back turned so that should he wish to stop at a certain shop not a word that he says can be heard. The baby frequently has a row of little plastic toys overhead; why could not the adult have a little plastic purse at the side for glasses and money! The pram often has a tray underneath; the wheelchair usually has no such device. A wheelchair has to have a pump. On a bicycle there is a place for it where it grips on; on a wheelchair there is nowhere to put it. If one could, the ideal thing would be to have two wheelchairs, one for out-of-doors and one for indoors, the latter padded and with the same loose covers as the rest of the sitting room that could be taken off and washed, and that matched the rest of the suite so not making one stick out like a sore thumb. For the outdoor model there needs to be some really way-out thinking – perhaps a rickshaw type of vehicle as seen in Singapore, where the driver or escort could be alongside like a motor bike and sidecar.

For the wheelchair pusher the most important point to remember is probably the kerb drill: 'up forwards, down backwards'.

Although the variety of wheelchairs is not great the range is slowly improving and there are a number of decisions which the disabled

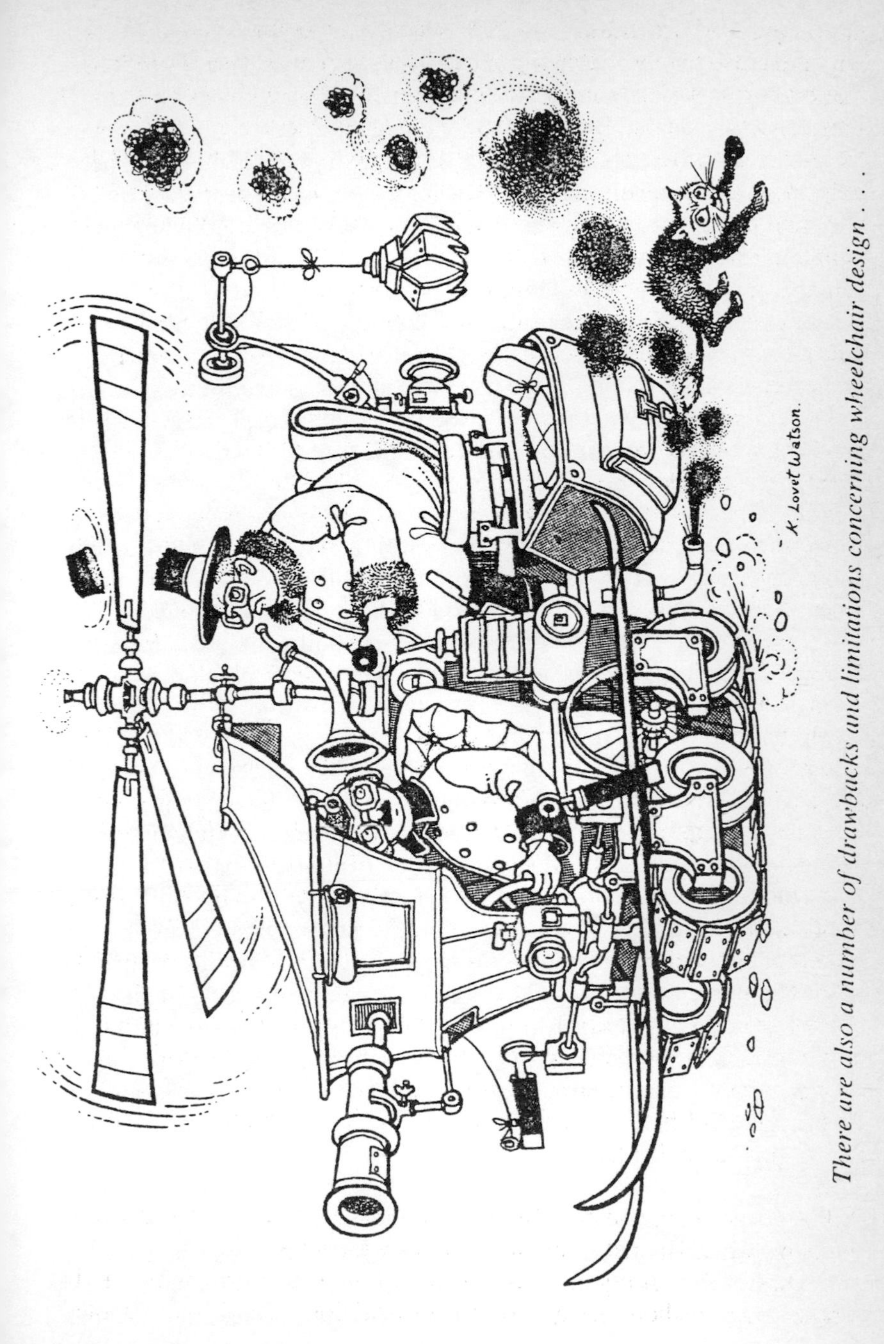

There are also a number of drawbacks and limitations concerning wheelchair design . . .

person will need to make. If the wheelchair is only required very occasionally, for example to take the person down a long approach footpath to the beach which can't be reached by car, then something like the very portable Buggy Major[3] could be a great asset. For more permanent use there are a variety of chairs available via the GP. These may be either for a helper to push or for the person to propel by use of the hands. For those people unable to use a self-propelled wheelchair then an electrically propelled version may be available. There is also a voucher scheme which the Government has introduced to allow some disabled people greater flexibility in the purchase of suitable wheelchairs, or they may be purchased privately. Some electric wheelchairs and scooters are not suitable for use both indoors and outdoors, so it is necessary to check whether the model is a dual-purpose one if it is required for use both inside and outside the home.

Shopping

Shopping expeditions need to be very well planned. It is not possible to engage in the luxury of a 'shopping ramble' in which you move from shop to shop picking up an odd article here and a few bits of grocery there. In general, people with MS find that they become very fatigued by such an approach. It is probably better to plan on going to one or two shops only for very specific items and to add further shopping only if the main objectives have been achieved without becoming overtired. The transport problems have been discussed in the previous section, and particular attention is drawn to the advantages of using a *Shopmobility* scheme where on offer.

For many people with MS mail order firms have proved a great assistance as with the sufferer who says: 'I mainly shop by mail order, very satisfactorily. I run a catalogue, it gives me an interest and keeps my brain ticking over having to do the paper work. It brings friends to see and pay me.' Other people rely on delivery services a great deal and on the help of friends. Relatives and friends may need to help the person with MS quite often with specific tasks such as the collection of the Disability Living Allowance,[4] Post Office and banking transactions.

Employment

A diagnosis of MS doesn't necessarily mean that a person becomes unable to work, and there are countless examples of MS sufferers who have continued to work in their chosen occupations – for example, as an architect, an air hostess working for an international airline company, a head teacher of a special school, a psychiatrist, a secretary, a company director, a telephonist/receptionist, an occupational therapist, a shop assistant, a research nurse, a University lecturer . . . Most people with MS would probably say that it is important to keep involved with a job for as long as possible. One MS sufferer, for example, managed to conceal his difficulties in walking for some time, but eventually his 'drunken' gait was too pronounced for him to remain as a police officer on patrol duty! In this case and in many similar cases people with MS have been able to transfer to lighter duties within the same occupational setting. The advice from one person with MS to somebody in their late twenties or early thirties who had just discovered they had MS was that they should 'Think ahead. You probably won't get a lot worse, but you might do, so if there's a possibility that you'll not be as good as you are now, then try and look ahead and train yourself or get yourself trained for something you can do even then, when you are not as agile as you are now.'[5] Planning ahead is clearly a key factor in the selection of an occupation. Physically tiring occupations and those involving finely coordinated movements may be found difficult, but as can be seen from the examples of people with MS who have continued to work in demanding occupations, it is often possible to find ways of coping – we heard in the last chapter of the MS sufferer who ran a business from his home with the aid of a Possum machine.

Sometimes, of course, the effects of MS do make it difficult for the person to cope with the demands of his or her job, and then a re-think is necessary. Often people with MS haven't actually told their employer about their condition, either because the doctors haven't confirmed it to them or because it isn't affecting their work and they are concerned that disclosing it would put their job in jeopardy. This is one of the difficult dilemmas often facing people with MS, but it usually resolves itself when the appearance of symptoms both confirms the MS and begs some explanation in the workplace. For example, the policeman with MS who appeared to be 'drunk on duty' would have been the subject of gossip and innuendo before his diagnosis was confirmed. But once his MS became known he would change from being 'the drunk in charge of the nick' to 'the copper with MS' who would be presented with a cheque for the MS Society, a result of the efforts of his colleagues in a sponsored half-marathon!

So, just as it is helpful for the doctor to discuss the diagnosis with the patient, when the diagnosis is clearly confirmed it is also helpful for the employee to be able to discuss his or her problems within the context of a supportive work environment. Constructive action can then be taken to the benefit of both employer and employee, such as a transfer to lighter duties. Such arrangements depend to a large extent, of course, on having a flexible and understanding employer, but the Disability Discrimination Act (1995) does place a requirement on employers to make reasonable changes to the workplace for a disabled person in employment to help overcome the practical effects of the employee's disability.[6] Other arrangements which have been found helpful have been to move to job-sharing or part-time work, in order to make life a bit easier; and early retirement is another option which has been taken by people in their later years.

If a person has been off sick with MS for a period of time, certain benefits become available (e.g. Incapacity Benefit). These are discussed in Chapter 8. But even then, this doesn't mean that some form of employment is entirely ruled out. For people in receipt of long-term Incapacity Benefit, for example, it is still possible to work for a limited number of hours each week (called 'therapeutic work') and to receive a certain level of payment if the work helps to improve or prevent or delay deterioration in the disease causing the incapacity for work. The work needs to be recommended by the doctor and agreed by the Benefits Agency, but in MS a limited amount of work of this nature is quite likely to be seen as appropriate since it will help to keep the person mentally alert, active and involved, all of which are beneficial elements in the management of MS. An example of 'therapeutic work' in practice can be seen in the case of a former lecturer who had to leave work because of his MS. He now receives Incapacity Benefit but has been able to work at the local University, helping with a research project for a few hours each week.

Holidays

In general, holidays tend to be organised for the able-bodied. Many guest-houses and hotels are quite inaccessible for the disabled. Brochures frequently present the most attractive picture of a holiday residence but fail to mention that there is a steep flight of steps to the entrance! There are a limited number of places with bedrooms and bathrooms on the ground floor, and although some hotels provide lifts these are not always sufficiently large to accommodate a wheelchair. Fortunately, there are some handbooks which give fuller information about such details.[7] There is still need, however, for a much more comprehensive range of booklets on this topic.

Many MS families have found that self-catering holidays are

successful provided that the accommodation is selected carefully. There are a number of bungalows available for hire and some specially converted holiday caravans. Occasionally, branches of the MS Society will have such accommodation available for their members. People with MS often find travelling tiring, however, and journeys will need to be carefully planned. Holiday routes need a liberal sprinkling of loo halts, in particular. (For a useful holiday planning aid see the *National Key Scheme Guide.* Under this scheme a number of toilets for the disabled throughout the UK have been fitted with special locks, keys for which may be obtained from the Local Authority or the Royal Association for Disability and Rehabilitation. A list of these toilets is available from RADAR.[8] There is also a route planning service (Route-finding and Access Maps Project, or RAMP) offered by the Disabled Motorists' Federation based at the National Mobility Centre, Banstead. See Chapter 8 for address.)

For those who like to travel abroad the travel agencies generally supply good information about facilities for the disabled. Air and sea travel is normally quite feasible and the disabled are generally very well looked after. Individual ferry/airlines will supply details of services offered and on air travel a free booklet is available – *Care in the Air* – offering advice for disabled travellers.[9]

Outside interests

It is very important that people with MS should not cut themselves off from outside interests and social events because of their handicap. In the early stages of the disease the MS sufferer may become embarrassed at having to leave parties early or at having to explain to acquaintances who have invited them to tea that they daren't come because there isn't a downstairs loo! For people in a wheelchair there is often a period when they feel quite embarrassed about their position. It is virtually impossible for someone in a wheelchair to slip in at the back quietly and unobserved! Most people, however, gradually come to the point where they accept that the advantages of increased mobility which a wheelchair brings far outweigh the initial disadvantages and embarrassments; but a few have to fight to reach this point of adjustment and require a good deal of support from family and friends.

Despite the difficulties people with MS often seem to manage to enter into an increasingly full social life. There are many leisure pursuits which can be engaged in despite physical handicap, and new interests are often developed through being a member of the local branch of the MS Society. Many MS sufferers manage to hold down full-time or part-time jobs or run the house. Others have found time for writing, painting, photography. Television, reading and music offer accessible areas for enjoyment and entertainment, and one woman in the local MS Society even booked a trip in an air balloon as an 80th birthday present!

Cinemas and theatres are not always accessible but most entertainment venues will try to accommodate disabled people where possible, so always ask! As far as sport is concerned, there are people with MS who enjoy swimming, riding and occasionally activities like table-tennis. Darts, chess and cards are all examples of games which people with MS can enjoy. The more strenuous aspects of gardening are often too fatiguing for someone with MS, but a great deal of gardening is possible, for example greenhouse gardening, raised flower bed or container gardening for the wheelchair bound and house plants. The book *Gardening is for Everyone*[10] has some very useful suggestions for the disabled gardener. For people who are interested in bird watching, the Royal Society for the Protection of Birds provides information on Nature Reserves suitable for people with disabilities.[11]

The person with MS faces very many problems and difficulties but these can frequently be overcome or modified if tackled with a resolute spirit. MS is often said to be characterised by a certain cheerfulness of mind or euphoria and it is true that MS sufferers do seem to bear the illness with a great degree of courage and positive thinking. Most people with MS, however, would probably object to the view that this is a feeling of well-being which stems from a lack of appreciation of the serious nature of the disease. MS sufferers are quite aware of the problems and can become quite depressed in the face of them. In general, though, by regarding the disease as a challenge they seem to find renewed strength to tackle their problems and in doing so provide a tremendous example of courage and tenacity to the more able-bodied among us. Indeed, people with MS often seem to live much fuller lives than able-bodied individuals and while coping with their immediate problems they are also hoping for the breakthrough in research which might indicate the cause of the disease and provide pointers to its cure.

The person with MS, therefore, tries to live a positive existence – an approach well illustrated by the following comments from two MS sufferers:

> During my schooldays I enjoyed the normal healthy ambitions to play football and cricket for England. These ambitions have now been replaced by a more down to earth one, which is to walk a

> straight line unassisted for fifteen yards. My main prayer is that this ambition is fulfilled as I am confident that I shall be able to build up fifteen yards to twice around the world.
>
> I believe in the power of positive thinking – don't look at what you can't do, concentrate on the things you can do. There is usually another way of doing things . . . be flexible. Treat it as a challenge – try and plan your day – work rest work rest principle – don't let people take over completely but be happy to let them help you when you are tired. Keep going. Get your priorities right.

MS can hit hard, but the MS sufferer can hit harder. It is surprising how effectively many people with MS manage to fight off the worst features of the disorder and find hidden strengths both in themselves and in members of their immediate family. It is interesting too how many MS sufferers find an amusing side to their illness. Stories told by MS sufferers themselves with a twinkle in their eye range from the married woman who trips into the arms of her milkman 'who didn't know she cared!' to the story of 'the uncontrollable leg':

> In bed . . . my leg would develop a violent uncontrollable spasm which often resulted in the knee causing a heavy blow to my wife's backside. I believe the leg, which at such times has a mind of its own, enjoys the experience, as changing bed positions has failed to totally eliminate such occurrences!

The ability to laugh at the symptoms of the disease is a great benefit to MS sufferers.

In summary, perhaps the three most important guiding principles for coping with MS are the three Ps: be Patient, Positive and Plan ahead. With such an approach coping becomes bearable, even enriching; and hoping, the forerunner of curing, keeps the spirit of optimism alive. One seventy-year-old woman who was a member of the local MS branch provides a marvellous example of this resolute spirit. She suffered from MS for thirty years and yet she kept alert and alive, looking after her ninety-year-old mother with the solicitous attention of a much younger person. Such a story must give hope to even the most faint-hearted.

6

Life-style: diet and exercise

We have seen how it is possible to cope effectively with a variety of problems which can arise in MS. In this chapter we will examine specific aspects of life-style in which it is possible for MS sufferers to make a positive contribution to their own well-being. In particular, we will look at the main components of a healthy, disease-resisting (and enjoyable) diet and at the sorts of exercises which physiotherapists feel are likely to be of benefit in MS.

General life-style measures

MS sufferers are familiar with the irritation of having to make *enforced* life-style changes – finding suitable forms of transport, using lifts instead of stairs, installing a downstairs loo – but there are plenty of changes you can introduce voluntarily by planning ahead in a positive manner. Since fatigue is often such a central problem in MS it is worth trying to plan your life so that you have a bit of time to recover in between activities:

> I try to plan my evenings out so that they don't come on top of each other. It's not always possible and you still want to do things on the spur of the moment – which I think is important. I'm determined not to let MS boss me around too much! But I also know my limitations and if I can space things out I always feel I can cope with things much better.

If you are a smoker it is worth giving serious consideration to cutting down or, preferably, giving up. Smoking constitutes a major health hazard. There is no evidence that smoking has any marked influence on the disease process in MS, but some symptoms may become worse for a short period immediately after smoking. Moreover, since some parts of your body are already impaired by MS, it's extremely important that you try to keep the rest in tip-top condition. Smoking will impede this aim by reducing the oxygen-carrying efficiency of the blood; by increasing the risk of circulation problems; and by impairing your level of general health in all sorts of ways. Evidence shows, for example, that smoking is the major cause of cancers of the lung, mouth and throat, and that smokers have a dramatically increased risk of developing heart disease and strokes when compared with non-smokers or with people who have given up the habit. On these issues the evidence is clear and unambiguous and is dealt with very fully in another book in this series which also gives detailed advice on how to quit smoking.[1] If you have tried different approaches to giving up smoking and are still finding difficulty because you have developed a high degree of physical dependence, you could try some form of nicotine replacement therapy (e.g. in chewing gum or skin patch form). Your GP will be able to advise you about this.

We have already discussed the importance of taking advantage where possible of labour-saving devices in the interests of conserving energy. But it is also important to keep as active as possible – we shall discuss ways of doing this in the section on exercise. In particular, because people with MS tend to be relatively immobile and unable to burn off excess calories by vigorous exercise, it's easy to become overweight. To counteract this tendency MS sufferers are likely to benefit from following some of the dietary advice discussed below, which involves plenty of healthy and enjoyable eating as well as some trimming of foods known to be linked to poor health.

If you want to check whether you are overweight you can do so by checking on the Body Mass Index (BMI) chart overleaf; or you can calculate you own BMI by using the following formula:

$$\text{weight (kg)} \div \text{height (m)}^2$$

Then you can see whether you are overweight by comparing your score with the following table:

BMI score	*Description*
less than 20	'underweight'
20–24.9	'acceptable'
25–29.9	'overweight'
30–40	'obese'
over 40	'severely obese'

So if you weigh 70 kg (11 stones) and are 1.73 m (5 ft 8 in) tall, you would have a BMI of 70 ÷ (1.73 × 1.73) = 23.4, which would put you in the 'acceptable' weight category.

These categories offer useful *general* guidance for both men and women. However, for older people, in their mid-sixties or above, there is some evidence that the recommended 'acceptable' category can creep up *just a little* bit into the 'overweight' category without creating too many problems. On the whole, being a little bit plumper at this stage in life doesn't seem to matter too much, but more careful weight control is, of course, still very important for people suffering from conditions such as diabetes or high blood pressure.

For people who are unable to take much exercise, as with MS sufferers, it also makes sense to prevent the plumpness becoming out of hand. Excessive weight is strongly associated with an increased risk of heart disease. In MS, obesity can also lead to an increase in sufferers' difficulties in walking, and create added problems for helpers lending a hand with walking and lifting or pushing the wheelchair! It's important to remember, however, that if you are overweight it's not a good idea to go on a crash diet. You should aim instead for a slow, steady weight loss – anything up to 1 kg (2 lb) a week would be reasonable. This can be achieved by eating a range of good, non-fattening foods (the sort described in the section on diet below) and by some deliberate trimming of the fattening extras, e.g. saving the crisps and chocolates as a treat and filling up on fruit and vegetables instead!

> It was my New Year's resolution to cut down my weight a bit. I was getting uncomfortably flabby! The main thing I did was to cut down on biscuits and I ate fruit instead of cake. I started eating a fig each day! I found out that figs were high in calcium, so they're good for protecting against osteoporosis (thinning of the bones). My doctor told me that this can become a problem in MS because we're not so active as other people. Anyway, I've lost 4 lb in about a month and I feel a lot more comfortable. I don't know about my bones but I drink lots of skimmed milk and try to eat foods high in calcium, like sardines and watercress. So with that and the figs something should be happening!

Diet in MS

As we have already seen, there is evidence that people with MS appear to have a deficiency in the level of polyunsaturated fat in their bodies. In particular, they appear to be deficient in the fatty acid known as linoleic acid, which is derived from vegetable oils such as sunflower seed oil. Lower levels of this fatty acid have been found in both the

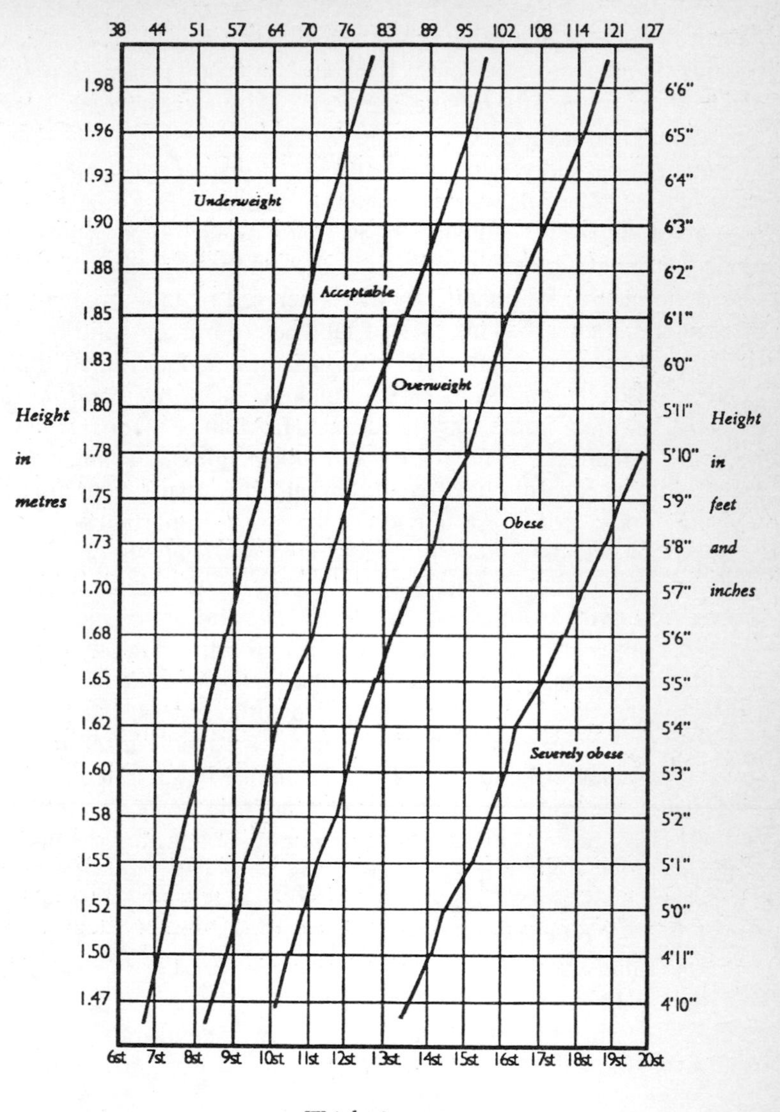

Body mass index (BMI) chart

myelin and in the blood of people with MS compared with groups of people without the disease.[2] Research has, therefore, been undertaken into the effects of increasing the intake of polyunsaturates in MS patients. But before we go on to look at some of this research in more detail, it will be helpful to take a closer look at the different types of fats we find in our food.

There are basically two types of fat – *saturated* and *unsaturated*. Most of the fats or oils we buy in the shops are, in fact, made up of a mixture of both. You can check how much of each type of fat is in a particular product by examining the labels on the container. Saturated fats are found predominantly in foods derived from animal sources, e.g. butter and cheese. This sort of fat tends to remain solid or semi-solid at room temperature, whereas unsaturated fats remain liquid. There are also two main kinds of unsaturated fats, *polyunsaturated* and *monounsaturated*. Some polyunsaturated fats can be made by our own bodies, but there are a few, the *essential fatty acids* (*omega*-6 and *omega*-3), that can only be obtained by ensuring a sufficient intake of relevant foods. For most purposes the most important source of omega-6 fatty acids is *linoleic acid*, found in vegetable oils such as sunflower seed oil.[3] Omega-3 fatty acids, on the other hand, are derived primarily from *alpha-linolenic acid* and are found in some vegetable oils such as soya bean and rapeseed oil, and in oily fish such as mackerel, herring, salmon and sardine.

Most of the diets which have been tried out in research studies have concentrated on increasing the consumption of polyunsaturated fat (especially omega-6) and decreasing the intake of saturated fats. The longest dietary trial was conducted by an American physician, Dr Swank. The study was initiated at the Montreal Neurological Institute in the late 1940s. A group of 144 patients were asked to follow a low fat diet and they were followed up for 34 years. Some patients (called 'good dieters') complied with the diet and others (the 'poor dieters') failed to comply and ate more fat than the diet prescribed. By the end of the study the good dieters were in better health than the poor dieters, with less deterioration in their MS and lower death rates. Unfortunately, the study did not satisfy the criteria usually required in medical research (e.g. the use of a controlled trial), and it is not possible to use the findings as a basis for firm conclusions. They do suggest, however, that fat levels may be implicated in MS, and Swank's work has led to considerable interest in the effects of fat intake on MS. His findings are also in line with general dietary advice, which indicates that most people would benefit from eating less saturated fat.

In the early 1980s another study of diet in MS was carried out at the Central Middlesex Hospital in London. The progress of MS patients was monitored after they had received nutritional advice to follow a diet high in polyunsaturates (especially the essential fatty acids, omega-3 and omega-6) and low in saturates, and to include foods high in anti-oxidant properties, such as fruit, nuts, vegetables and wholemeal cereals. Again, the study did not include a control group but relied upon dividing the patients arbitrarily into a group of patients who adhered fairly closely to the diet and one in which they complied less well. Despite the limitations in the design of the study, the findings were encouraging in that those who followed the dietary advice closely tended on average to remain neurologically more stable over the three years of the study than those who kept to the diet less rigorously.

A number of other research studies have examined the effects of polyunsaturated supplements using controlled, double blind designs. The results show a distinct trend in favour of the groups treated with the omega-6 linoleic acid supplement, patients in these groups showing a reduced level of severity of MS attacks compared with the controls. When the data from three of these major dietary studies were combined, the results were even more clear cut, with the treated groups showing a significant reduction in the progression of the disease.[4] A promising trend in favour of a group treated with omega-3 linolenic acid supplement was also observed in a trial involving 312 patients, carried out under the supervision of Professor Bates at the University of Newcastle.

The evidence so far is, therefore, encouraging on the value of using polyunsaturated dietary supplements in MS. What is also very clear is that both omega-6 and omega-3 polyunsaturates bring important health benefits over and above their possible advantages in MS. In particular, they have important roles to play in the prevention of heart disease. For example, omega-6 fatty acids help to lower cholesterol, and the omega-3 variety have been found to help in preventing the blood from clotting and in controlling high blood pressure. So the use of polyunsaturates in the diet is clearly something that can be recommended.

> I use a polyunsaturated margarine, spread thinly on bread, and sunflower oil for cooking. I also take Naudicelle Plus capsules as a supplement, the ones made from Oil of Evening Primrose and Fish Oil. I've been taking them for years and my MS has kept pretty

stable. I know the research evidence isn't entirely clear-cut, but they won't do me any harm and they might be doing me a lot of good!

Another line of dietary research has been concerned with the role of the anti-oxidant vitamins in counteracting MS. It seems possible that chemical agents in the body called 'free radicals', which encourage the oxidization of fats and are already implicated in a number of diseases (including cancer), may also be involved in some way in MS. The evidence is so far very limited, but if the theory is correct it makes sense to try to counteract the free radicals by eating food containing anti-oxidant vitamins, which help 'mop up' the free radicals in our bodies.[5] Moreover, since the foods in which anti-oxidant vitamins are present are beneficial to health in all sorts of other ways, they can be eaten in the certain knowledge they will be doing you good! The anti-oxidant vitamins are:

- *beta-carotene* (a form of vitamin A) – found in green, yellow and orange vegetables, and not destroyed by cooking. Particularly high quantities can be obtained from carrots and dark green vegetables such as spinach. Also contained in a wide range of fruits and vegetables, e.g. apricots, mangoes, sweet melons, red peppers, broccoli, watercress and lettuce;
- *vitamin C* – found in a wide variety of fruit and vegetables, especially citrus fruits, blackcurrants, strawberries, guavas, broccoli, greens, parsley, peppers and new potatoes. Cooked fruits and vegetables will lose some of their vitamin content;
- *vitamin E* – found in vegetable oils such as sunflower seed oil, wholemeal cereals, leafy vegetables and nuts, and not destroyed by cooking;
- *selenium* – a trace element found in cereals, fish and nuts.

While dealing with vitamins it is also worth repeating that vitamin B_{12} has been found to be of particular benefit to people with MS, and can be taken orally or prescribed in injection form by your doctor. It is also found in yeast extract and quite often in breakfast cereals.

To summarise the findings on diet we can say that the person with MS should aim generally to eat a healthy diet by:

- eating a wide variety of foods and particularly foods with anti-oxidant properties;
- keeping low on fats and using polyunsaturated rather than saturated fat;

- watching for the 'hidden fat' in foods like biscuits, cakes and crisps;
- choosing lean cuts of meat and low-fat cheese;
- grilling rather than frying;
- drinking skimmed or semi-skimmed milk;
- keeping low on sugar and salt;
- keeping to a moderate intake of alcohol (it sometimes seems to have a stronger than normal effect in people with MS!);
- eating plenty of fruit and vegetables (at least 5 portions a day);
- eating oily fish such as mackerel, sardines and herring;
- eating plenty of starchy foods like breakfast cereals, bread, potatoes and pasta;
- choosing wholemeal foods (e.g. bran, wholemeal bread) to help prevent constipation.

You should find this sort of diet enjoyable as well as healthy. Together with the sort of exercises described in the next section it should enable you to keep in good trim!

Exercises and MS

Physiotherapy is a major contributor to the maintenance of fitness for people with MS. It is important that each person is assessed by a qualified physiotherapist and for treatment to be tailored to individual needs. In this way fatigue can be avoided, progress monitored and problems dealt with as they arise. The community physiotherapist can be of particular value in providing this kind of support. There are a few suggestions for exercise for MS sufferers which are of *general* relevance, however, and these are described below. But first we must look at some of the reasons why exercise is useful.

Why is exercise important?

Exercise is essential to keep our bodies in good working order! In particular, it will help you maintain a healthy heart and good blood circulation. It increases the supply of oxygen in the blood, helps increase your energy levels and stamina, reduces stiffness and increases suppleness in the joints. It also helps lower cholesterol, reduce stress and promote a general feeling of well-being. So there are lots of reasons for trying to exercise the body as much as possible, whatever the degree of disability. The range of possible activities will obviously be affected by the degree of severity of the disabilities caused by MS, but even in the most severe cases it is usually possible to find a number of exercises which will have some beneficial effects.

Some general advice on exercise

It is essential for people with MS to try to maintain a good range of movement in their joints. The general advice is to keep moving as much as possible. For those who can manage activities like walking, cycling and swimming, these are excellent forms of exercise. In fact any form of exercise which helps keep the joints supple and increase oxygen consumption is usually beneficial. For people who have a more restricted range of movement, however, there are still plenty of possible exercises. Remember, however, that you need to listen to your body when you are exercising. If you begin to feel tired or to experience discomfort, stop straight away. Getting over-fatigued can defeat the object of the exercise!

> I find it useful to have a rest in between doing things, but I also remind myself when it's a bit of a struggle: 'If I don't use it there's more chance I'll lose it!' So I keep moving all the parts I can, and I'm still going quite well, even if I do say so myself. I'm walking more than I did, and I still do most of the shopping and cooking.

Of particular importance for wheelchair users are exercises involving the hips and knees, which can tend to become rather rigid and stiff if preventive action isn't taken. In particular, knees can become fixed in a flexed, bent-up position. If your joints won't move too easily by themselves you could try to get them moving with the help of your hands, or with someone else's assistance. This sort of 'passive' movement can help keep your joints from becoming too stiff or fixed from disuse, and help prevent contractures. By actively seeking out your own ways of improving your body's mobility, and by following the physiotherapists' advice on exercise, you may find that your potential range of movements is greater than you imagined.[6]

> The fingers of my right hand were bent in like a claw and I had a lot of difficulty in getting them to move at all. So I used to pull them back and 'unclaw' my hand as much as possible. If I was sitting down watching television I'd exercise my hand, and each finger separately. I don't know whether it was my exercises that did it but after several months I found that my hand was getting less clawed, and I can now stretch the fingers out a bit.

Practising a range of movements in your joints, like lifting your knees up and then stretching your legs out (or getting someone to do these exercises for you), will also help in stretching the muscles. This, in turn, can help prevent muscle spasms and also to relieve the pain experienced from them. You could even try some exercises in bed, e.g. bending your knees up, rolling from side to side, lying on your tummy and trying to bring your heels up towards your bottom.

Another common problem in MS which can be helped by exercise is that of poor balance and coordination. Because of balance problems people with MS are understandably reluctant to try standing without support. But with a strategically placed grab handle, walking frame or helper as a safety net, standing unsupported or with minimal support for a short time each day can be an excellent form of exercise. It helps strengthen the postural muscles and improve balance. Similarly, sitting upright for a short time with as straight a back as you can manage without support is another good exercise for posture. Horse-riding is one activity which has been found beneficial for balance by a number of people with MS; others find that swimming is particularly helpful (provided the water is neither too cold nor too hot). One member of the local branch of the MS Society (a strong swimmer before he developed MS) found that swimming was still a particularly good exercise for him. Despite his MS, he regularly used to test his balance and coordination by climbing up to the diving board and performing superb dives into the pool! Not an exercise to be recommended as a general rule in MS, of course, but it does illustrate the importance of looking at each individual's strengths and weaknesses and planning exercises appropriately and imaginatively.

For people who have to spend a lot of time in a sitting position the back and shoulders can become stooped, breathing become shallow, pressure increase on the abdomen, bladder, back and bottom. All this can result in considerable discomfort and pain. Postural exercises can help with these problems, especially yoga, which some MS sufferers have found very helpful.[7] If you're in a wheelchair or sit in an ordinary chair for long periods of time it's also a good idea to lift yourself up in the chair every half-hour or so (or get someone to help you) to relieve your bottom from the constant pressure of sitting down. Without such relief it is very easy for the skin to develop sores.

> I push myself up in the chair and move my position quite frequently. I twiddle my toes as well and do 'up-and-down' dancing movements with my feet and legs as a sort of exercise to music!

> And when I stand at the kitchen sink I hold on to the sink and pretend I'm a ballet dancer. I bend my legs a bit and stretch them out to the side.

So-called 'weight-bearing' exercises – the ones in which your joints are holding up the weight of your body or parts of your body – are particularly good for helping to counteract osteoporosis (thinning or weakening of the bones resulting from depletion in calcium in the body). Standing and walking are, therefore, particularly good exercises from this point of view. If you can do this in sunlight, so much the better as sunlight helps our body absorb calcium.[8] There is also some evidence that exposure to sunlight (but not *hot sun*, since excessive heat can lead to temporary weakness and increased fatigue) may be of general benefit in MS. This may well relate to the role of sunlight in the production of vitamin D and in the release of the antioxidant vitamin A, but further research is required to establish the relationships more clearly.

Apart from exercising, stopping smoking, and eating foods rich in calcium, hormone replacement therapy (HRT) is also a very effective way of preventing osteoporosis in middle-aged and older women. In addition, there is evidence from a small pilot study carried out at King's College Hospital in London that HRT may have beneficial effects on MS symptoms. Taken together with the evidence that women with MS often tend to feel particularly well during pregnancy and to have fewer MS episodes, there does seem to be some indication that hormonal factors may have a part to play in MS. Again, further research is required to establish the extent to which such factors are implicated in the disease process.

Hydrotherapy (exercise carried out in a pool of warm water) is sometimes found to be of benefit in MS, but for quite a number of people the warmth of the water has the result of inducing post-therapy fatigue. It's certainly worth a try if your physiotherapist offers you a few trial sessions, but the best advice (here your physio will certainly concur) is to be guided by your own body as to whether it is working for you. Swimming, or doing exercises, in an ordinary swimming pool in which the water is reasonably warm could be even better. A lot of swimming pools are a bit on the cool side for MS sufferers, but you'll sometimes find that the smaller (children's) pools are heated to a more comfortable temperature; and many of these are just deep enough for you to be able to carry out a few useful exercises on your own or with the help of a friend. What is so morale boosting about being in water is that the buoyancy enables you to do all sorts of exercises that seem impossible on dry land!

> I can't walk very easily in normal circumstances, but when I get in the water I can lift my knees up to amazing heights! All my movements seem much freer, and with the floats I can lie back in the water and relax . . . it's paradise!

Pain relief

As we have seen, people who are not very mobile and tend to spend prolonged periods sitting down often develop weak postural muscles (e.g. those in the back and abdomen). This can result, in turn, in back pain sufficiently severe to require treatment. Ordinary pain relieving drugs can be of help in this situation, but it is also possible to reduce the pain by the application of heat, by using a cold compress, by using ultra-sound treatment, or by the use of a transcutaneous electrical nerve stimulator (known as a *TENS* machine). As far as the use of heat or cooling treatment is concerned, it is worth trying a hot or cold compress pack (the type often used for sporting injuries), or, for heat treatment alone, an electric heat pad. These are sold quite widely in chemists or shopping catalogues and are often quite sufficient to relieve the discomfort. Care must be taken when using treatments of this sort as it is possible to burn yourself, especially if your MS has led to altered skin sensation. Ultra-sound treatment is available via the physiotherapist, as is treatment by a *TENS* machine (although this machine is often lent to patients for home use). If this form of treatment is found to be particularly helpful, *TENS* machines may also be purchased privately.[9] There are also several alternative therapies, such as acupuncture and reflexology, which have found favour as pain relieving/relaxing therapies with a number of MS sufferers.

In summary, we cannot so far cure MS by attention to life-style measures of the sort discussed in this chapter, but it is possible to improve the *quality of life* very considerably by taking care about what we eat and how we exercise our bodies. With this approach to fighting MS we can enjoy a better quality of life at the moment and keep ourselves in shape for a better future to come.

7

How can the MS Society help?

Most people have heard of MS and often know someone with it; for many people diagnosed with the condition, however, it comes as a bolt from the blue. There is a general assumption that there will be an organisation to help, but the MS Society is less well known than the disease. Every month hundreds of people, many of them newly diagnosed, make their first contact with the Society to ask for information or help through the national MS Helpline service (see Chapter 8). Often this will be all they need at the time, and it may be months or even years before they contact the Society again. This is as it should be; the Society does not force its advice or help on anyone. Most first-time callers will receive a basic information pack, and although it includes an invitation to opt for further mailings or become a member, there is no pressure to do so. The Helpline and the rest of the Society's services are available to anyone with MS as and when they need them.

The Society has tens of thousands of members, some of whom join directly through its headquarters, in London, while many join one of the 370 local branches covering Scotland, Northern Ireland, Wales and England. Understandably, some people do not want to acquire the 'label' of having MS through participating in a group, do not want to define themselves as disabled, or are apprehensive about meeting people with MS who have advanced or severely disabling forms of the disease. But becoming a member of the Society does not require participation in group meetings, and mailings from the branches and headquarters will keep members in touch with important developments as they take place. The Society aims to 'be there' whenever it is needed for the whole community of people with MS and their carers. Being a member, whether or not an active one, is a gesture of mutual concern for all the 80,000 people who live with the same uncertainties.

Increasingly, the MS Society is able to offer people whose choice is not to join one of the local groups other ways of participating in its work. The high quality life-style magazine *MS Matters* was launched in 1995, as the periodical 'for people living with MS'. A positive and vivacious publication, it aims to be a good and interesting read for everyone, and puts the emphasis on living, rather than being overwhelmed by MS. It is published every two months, and always includes ways of responding to the information and news it carries. Thus questionnaires may invite personal accounts of achievements or setbacks in living with MS, in employment, with the health services or in using the Society's own services. The responses are read carefully and help to shape the work the Society does on behalf of the MS community, whether in lobbying for improved benefits, better healthcare, or its own planning. *MS Matters* is sent to all members, and from 1996 has also been available, on subscription, to non-members.

For people who left school after the Information Technology revolution began, using the Internet or other ways of communicating by computer is routine, and as the technology advances it will become easier for everyone. In 1995 the MS Society started its own experimental Internet site. Interest was so great that a year later it was running a site on the World Wide Web on behalf of all 34 MS societies throughout the world, called WoMS – the World of MS. This carries news updates and most of the Society's main publications. The address of the site is *http://www.ifmss.org.uk* For readers wishing to contact the Society directly via e-mail, with queries or requests for information, the address is *info@mssociety.org.uk* There are also a number of public MS bulletin boards which come and go on the Internet, though the items of information and expressions of opinion that find their way onto these are often not checked for accuracy or authenticity.

Local branches

The Society is one of Britain's largest charities, set up in 1953 by Richard Cave, himself a carer. Self-help and mutual support have always been among its ways of working, in which the local branches play a key role. Simply sharing the experience of living with this mysterious condition, discovering that you are not alone, and learning how other people manage their symptoms, can be a powerful therapy. The branches serve this purpose first and foremost, and are the front line in providing help locally. Each one is unique, as reflected in the work they do. All but a few are run entirely by volunteers, many of whom are people with MS and carers – only proper in a self-help organisation! The style and extent of their work, the success of their fund-raising, and the scope of their resources reflect this. Some branches restrict their meetings to a monthly information meeting and social gathering, while others have a wide array of different services and activities. Separate meetings for people with varying interests, such as newly diagnosed groups or young people's groups, are run by some branches. Counselling to help deal with the emotional and psychological effects of MS is an important service offered by branches, complemented by three telephone counselling services supported by the Society in London, the Midlands and Scotland. Other branches run training courses on learning to cope with MS; some keep in touch through telephone networks; many produce their own entertaining and original newsletters. Frequently, branches invite outside speakers to talk about research, symptom management, therapies or the Society's work.

Complementing the work of the local health and Social Services is an important role for the branches. In many areas they offer regular physiotherapy sessions, transport, or visiting services. A number of larger branches run day centres offering a remarkable range of services, and like most branches see transport as one of the most important. Some manage their own specially adapted holiday facilities, while others organise and may meet the cost of family or group holidays in Britain or abroad. The Northern Ireland branch of the Society, from its base in Belfast, offers all these services and more. Increasingly, the branches work in partnership with their local health and social care providers, to try to ensure that the statutory services are organised in a way that truly reflects the needs of people with MS. As the organisations that have by far the greatest experience of managing the disease and caring for those affected by it, the Society's branches are increasingly recognised as a source of expertise and advice.

It is a basic requirement of charity law that resources are used equitably. This means that it is not necessary to be a member of a branch to receive help, and that the branches of the Society, like the headquarters, try to offer help to everyone in need; the only qualification is that of having MS or being a carer. But the Society's resources are, of course, limited, and it is not in a position to provide for all needs. An important facet of being part of a branch is the sense of companionship that it can bring. This is summed up by one member:

> My friends and others didn't understand how I felt, and I couldn't explain. I felt odd, an outcast, embarrassed. Then by chance my sister-in-law (who is a health visitor) put me in touch with the Society. I felt at ease with the people I met in the local branch, they accepted me as I am, I could identify with them. Joining the MS Society has given me great pleasure and a sense of belonging, as well as the most useful information of all.

One of the Society's unique services is its network of nine respite centres and holiday homes throughout the UK. Each has its own distinctive character, from the purpose-built Brambles near Gatwick, Leuchie near Edinburgh (run on behalf of the Society by an order of nuns, in a magnificent stately home), to Danygraig in South Wales (run as a joint venture between the Society, the health service and local authority Social Services. The homes are run for the Society by committed professional staff, but are managed by volunteers. They give the interests of their guests, and the provision of high quality services, the utmost priority. But they have high staff-to-guest ratios and are expensive to run. A large proportion of their costs is met by the Society centrally, but several of the centres have specialist staff whose work includes negotiating with various funders a financial contribution to the cost of a guest's stay.

It is easy to slip into the frame of mind whereby people with MS are defined by *dis*ability rather than by *ability*. The dramatic and arresting advertising undertaken by the Society itself in the late 1980s and early 1990s has been held partly responsible for this, but the fact is that the public at large has stereotyped images it applies to *every* medical condition. An important part of the Society's current work is to emphasise ability, through drawing attention in the media to the achievements of people with MS, as well as in publicity and fund-raising on behalf of the charity. It also supports special projects that embody this principle, such as Multiple Challenge, which originated in the Whitbread Round Britain yacht races. A professional yachtmaster whose mother suffered from MS provided the inspiration for crews of people with MS to enter these extremely demanding races, and not only to come well up the field, but also to raise money for the Society through sponsorship.

Extensive though the MS Society is, it is not the only source of help. Around the country there are several dozen therapy centres – independent charities that used to be part of a national organisation that closed in the 1980s. These centres emphasise self-management of MS, but offer a variety of therapies including physiotherapy, counselling and hyperbaric oxygen treatment. Where this is offered the therapy centres now operate a code of safe practice for its use.

The relationship between the therapy centres and the MS Society branches varies locally; some operate shared services or provide joint information, while virtually all have members in common. There are also a number of smaller national charities interested in different aspects of MS, such as the education of health professionals, aspects of research, information services, long-term care and complementary or alternative therapies. The MS Society takes the view that where organisations share the common goal of working for the interests of people with MS, it should collaborate with them to the best possible effect, and not take a rigid view on the right way to do things.

For many people with MS, their most pressing need is information, both to keep abreast of the advances in research and treatment that are now beginning to appear at an increasing rate, and to help them to manage the disease instead of letting it manage them. *MS Matters* incorporates a regular update on biomedical science (but written in plain English!), and the Society produces a series of information leaflets to explain the facts about MS as well as aspects of living with the condition. An important part of this is trying to explain MS to the general public through an active media relations programme, and the Society is recognised as the media's authoritative source of information, whether or not its name is quoted. It aims to look dispassionately at the evidence for claimed treatments, examining the facts rather than the speculation. This is sometimes an unpopular position, but for people whose only certainty is all to often uncertainty, it provides a strongpoint amidst the blizzard of claims and counterclaims. The Society is dogmatic on only two aspects of treatment claims, whether drugs, diets or other ideas. First, if people are not being exploited or harmed, they should be free to try whatever makes them feel better, even if the scientific evidence is not yet available to prove or disprove a claim (people with MS are almost all adult by definition, and must be free to make their own choices). But, second, it strongly advocates properly conducted clinical trials as the only means of testing treatments, and has a long record of supporting trials for this purpose.

Funding research

The Society is by far the largest funder of research on MS in the UK, and one of the largest in the world. At any one time it is supporting fifty or more projects in different hospitals and universities throughout the country. These range from basic science such as cell biology, which aims to explain the underlying processes of MS, to applied research on aspects of treatment or symptom management that are hoped to make a difference in the short term. MS is now known to be a complex disease involving the interplay of several factors – environment, genetic susceptibility, and the metabolism of the central nervous system. As a result, medical scientists expect that finding an answer will be just as lengthy a process as it has been for other complex disorders, and that if there were a single obvious causal factor it would have been found by now.

For many years it was doubted whether light would ever dawn. But in 1995 the first treatment for the underlying processes of the disease was licensed in the UK and Europe: an interferon manufactured by the pharmaceutical company Schering, and marketed under the name Betaferon – see Chapter 2. Its development, which had been going on for over a decade, was in the end possible because of the pioneering work on magnetic resonance imaging carried out at the Institute of Neurology in London, and funded by the MS Society.

When first introduced, Betaferon was a very costly treatment – at 1996 prices, about £10,000 per patient per year. It was argued by some policymakers that this was too high a price to pay for a compound which did not produce dramatic results, but simply alleviated the relapses which would get better anyway. In its role as a lobbying body, the MS Society mounted a campaign to ensure that this and other drugs shown to have benefit would be prescribed and their costs met through the NHS, just as for any other condition. It argued that scarcely anything had been spent on MS over the lifetime of the NHS, and that to deny the new treatments now would be an affront to natural justice. The Society did not demand that the treatments should be available ad lib, but within the limits which trials had shown to be effective. At the national level this was accepted, but since decisions on prescribing are made by individual doctors, and on purchasing by local health authorities, the argument often had to take place all over again, though this time with the backing of health ministers and the written guidance of the Department of Health.

In the run-up to the licensing of the first treatment, the media had been over enthusiastic in their claims, describing the interferons as 'wonder drugs', which they plainly were not. People with MS were becoming confused about the facts, and turning to one organisation after another to try to get clear information. The Society, again following the line that everything should be done to reduce uncertainty, got together with all the smaller MS charities providing an information service to produce a common fact-sheet on the new drugs. By the time Betaferon was licensed, virtually everyone with MS, together with all neurologists and many GPs, had received this. As a result they were able to take a calm and rational view of the potential of the treatment, and much of the anxiety and false hope evaporated. The charities have continued to work together on this, and plan to produce further common information on the treatments and aspects such as clinical trials as they come into the pipeline.

Joining the Society

So, how do people (sufferers, their family and friends, or anyone else) become members of the Multiple Sclerosis Society? If local branch members are not already known, or you are unable to find a telephone number for the local branch in the phone book, then contact the head office of the Society, which will supply the address of your nearest local branch secretary. The subscription to the Society is very small, and is paid direct to the local branch. The address and other important details will be found in the next chapter.

8

Other sources of practical help outside the family

The purpose of this book has been to show how it is possible to come to terms, and cope with, a disability. For many MS sufferers the great challenge is to retain their independence, but as Chapters 4 and 5 suggest, in doing so there is an in-built contradiction in terms – namely, that in order best to retain that precious independence, the sufferer must be willing and able to make use of the very many areas of practical help which exist outside the immediate family and friends. In this chapter we shall concentrate on the types of help available outside the family.

In general, the most successful adjustment is made by thinking out the problems involved in leading the kind of life you want to lead, and then looking for solutions. Of all the problems, probably the most common and frustrating to the person who is disabled is that of fatigue. The first thing, therefore, is to discover easier and less tiring ways of doing the essential everyday things, so that energy and resources may be saved for doing those things which, from personal choice, make life most worthwhile.

To overcome a practical problem, different people need different levels and forms of assistance. Aids are not necessarily the solution to every problem, and the individual may often be reluctant to accept the necessity for such an aid, feeling that its use is an admission of some sort of defeat. However, many people have found that the use of appropriate aids entirely changes their life-style – and often the simplest aid is the best. We cannot hope to give detailed specialist advice on the range of equipment and the various forms of financial and practical assistance available. This chapter, however, points the reader to the sources from which specialized help and advice is available. Also included are the addresses of agencies which exist to enable the disabled person to continue to be active in special hobbies, or find new ones, thus filling the need for opening up new horizons and making new friends. Finally, a list of helpful reference books is provided to supplement those included in the main body of the text.

First points of contact

The General Practitioner

The very first point of contact will, in most cases, be the General Practitioner. Many benefits from the Social Services Department depend on the referral or recommendation of GPs, so they should be kept acquainted with any changes in the condition of the patient. The GP can make arrangements for the disabled person to be contacted regarding such essential assistance as Home Helps, the Health Visitor, the Community Nurse, and either the GP or the hospital consultant can arrange for the loan of aids such as wheelchairs or walking sticks. Wheelchairs can also be obtained on short-term loan from agencies such as the Red Cross Society. Many people with disabilities will receive regular visits from the Community Nurse, although the regularity of such visits will obviously depend upon the nature of the person's condition. Medical aid which might include hospital treatment, or home physiotherapy or chiropody, can also be arranged through liaison between the GP and the hospital.

Hospital

The MS sufferer may be referred to the Physiotherapy Department for assessment and advice about mobility and daily living problems. A suitable home exercise programme may be recommended and provision for walking aids will be made where appropriate. Arrangements can also be made to supply a wheelchair where necessary, and the Occupational Therapist may be asked to carry out an assessment of daily needs on such matters as kitchen and bathroom facilities. Arrangements will be made for the provision of appropriate aids and adaptations to the home.

The Social Services Department

The Chronically Sick and Disabled Persons' Act (1970)[1] gave details of some of the services that should be available to the disabled, and required local authorities to identify the disabled in their areas and to provide information on the services available to them. The Carers (Recognition and Services) Act (1996) also gives the right to *carers* to have *their* needs assessed when the person they are caring for is being considered for community care services. Contact with the Social Services will normally begin with a visit from the Local Authority Social Worker or Community Occupational Therapist. But whether or not such contact has been made, information and advice about a number of services is available through the staff of the Social Service Department, who liaise with other departments. The community care services may vary slightly between different authorities but they may include the following:

1 Practical assistance in the home, including provision or loan of special aids and structural alterations to assist mobility about the home and independence in general.
2 Structural alterations to homes, such as the widening of doors and construction of ramps, as well as the provision of walking aids and aids for bathroom and kitchen; also such major items as hydraulic hoists, adjustable tilting beds and lifts can all be grant assisted or provided by local authorities. Electronic support systems[2] are also available, and severely disabled patients are advised to make enquiries about these, since evidence suggests that many people who could use them to their advantage know little or nothing about them.
3 Help from Occupational Therapists and Physiotherapists may sometimes be available via the Social Services Department as well as the hospital. They can be contacted through the GP or Social Worker. The Occupational Therapist assesses the practical needs of disabled people to live and work as normally as possible, operating on a visiting basis and giving advice on equipment and necessary alterations. The physiotherapist helps to maintain bodily movement as far as possible, and will in some cases make regular home visits.
4 Recreational and educational facilities: these vary among authorities, but many provide Day Centres and can give information on special courses, adult education centres and other facilities provided by voluntary organisations.
5 Assistance with the provision of telephones for those who are at risk or isolated from friends and neighbours – information is also available from British Telecom on special adaptations for the disabled, particularly the hard of hearing.
6 Provision of television and radio for those isolated from social contact.
7 Home Help Service: this can be provided for as little or as much time per week as is thought necessary, and the cost of this help

with housework, cooking and shopping is based on a means test assessment.

8 Holidays: a number of special publications exist dealing with holidays for the disabled,[3] and local authorities or the MS Society can give financial assistance in providing holidays.

9 Parking discs: most authorities provide special Orange badges enabling more convenient parking for the disabled.

10 Attendance at and help in getting to Day Centres, Luncheon Clubs and Social Clubs – these are often run by voluntary organisations, but the Social Worker can put you in contact with them.

11 Meals on Wheels – provision of meals can be provided by the Social Services Department on direct application.

12 Housing: although local authorities have limited resources for the housing of the disabled, many people can be moved to housing more suitable for their needs, and some authorities provide purpose-built houses and flats. In general rehousing is indicated where access to the bathroom or toilet is difficult, or where it is necessary for a person to be housed on one floor level.

13 Home chiropody treatment is sometimes available.

Disablement Employment Adviser

Disablement Employment Advisers work from local Jobcentres. They are specially trained to help disabled people resettle into suitable employment, and have close contact with employers, doctors, hospital and Social Services. Their aim is to help disabled people achieve their maximum potential for employment, and they can be a source of practical help and morale boosting for the newly diagnosed sufferer who can see little or no working future ahead.

Benefits and allowances

For most of us the complicated range of benefits and allowances available is a frightening maze, and rather than become lost in its bureaucratic intricacies or face possible disappointment, people will often prefer to do without. There are, however, many benefits which can considerably help improve the quality of life for the disabled person and his/her family. Leaflets and advice can be obtained from any Social Security office, and particularly helpful are the leaflets entitled 'Which Benefit?' (FB2) and 'Social Security Benefit Rates'

(NI 196). The telephone number of your local office will be found in the telephone directory under Benefits Agency. For general advice you can also call the freephone Benefit Enquiry Line (BEL) for people with disabilities on 0800 88 22 00. There are also three other very important sources of information for discovering what current benefits are available, who is eligible for them and how to set about obtaining them:

1. The Disability Rights Handbook

Published by: The Disability Alliance ERA,
1st Floor East, Universal House
88–94 Wentworth Street, London E1 7SA
Tel. 0171–247 8776

This is an annual publication, updated each year, and is a fully comprehensive guidebook to rights, benefits and services available to disabled people and their families, making it easy to discover which benefits you are entitled to, and showing clearly the procedure for obtaining them. It should be available in your local library or Citizens' Advice Bureau. The Disability Alliance Educational and Research Association will also offer advice on social security benefits by phone (see page 82).

2. Disablement Information and Advice Lines (DIAL) UK

Head Office: DIAL (UK) Park Lodge,
St Catherine's Hospital, Tickhill Road,
Balby, Doncaster DN4 8QN
Tel. 01302 310123

This is a nationwide telephone information and advice service, manned by trained disabled volunteers, and able to give thorough up-to-date advice and information on benefits, allowances and services. There are over 75 local support groups throughout the UK. Contact the above address for your nearest group.

3. Citizens' Advice Bureaux

National Association of Citizens' Advice Bureaux (NACAB)
Middleton House, 115–123 Pentonville Road,
London N1 9LZ
Tel. 0171 833 2181

You should be able to find the number of your local Citizens' Advice

Bureau in the telephone directory, but in case of difficulty NACAB has details of all CABs. These will offer help and advice on a whole range of problems, including difficulties in dealing with benefit entitlements.

The leaflet Which benefit?, issued by the Benefits Agency and available from your local Social Security Office, gives details of most Social Security and NHS benefits. Enquiries to the local Social Security office may be necessary in order to check on the availability of benefits in individual cases, but the main benefits are as follows:

1 Disability Living Allowance: a tax-free benefit for people who need help with personal care or with getting around or both. It provides three rates of help for Care needs and two for Mobility needs.
2 Attendance allowance: a tax-free benefit available to people aged 65 or over who need help with personal care and have needed looking after day and/or night for at least six months.
3 Invalid Care Allowance: a non-contributory allowance for men and single women of working age who have to stay at home to care for a severely disabled relative who is getting attendance or disabled living allowance. The allowance is liable to tax.
4 Disability Working Allowance: a tax-free (but means-tested) benefit for people who have an illness or disability that puts them at a disadvantage in getting a job, and are starting to work or are already working.
5 Assistance with fares to work: for severely disabled persons who are registered as disabled and who, for reasons of their disability, are unable to use public transport for all or part of their journey to and from work, resulting in extra travel costs. Claims should be made through the Disablement Employment Adviser at the Jobcentre.
6 Family Credit: this is a means-tested Social Security benefit for families on low wages who have children.
7 Free dental treatment, free prescriptions, vouchers for glasses: families or people on low incomes or receiving income support, and some disabled people, may be eligible for assistance. For full details check in the *Disability Rights Handbook.*
8 Housing Benefit: this is a means-tested benefit which gives help with paying rent. Details can be obtained from council offices.

9 Income Support: this is a means-tested benefit for people on low incomes. Extra financial help may also be available in certain circumstances through the discretionary Social Fund. Check with your local Social Security office for details.

10 Incapacity Benefit: available for people unable to work because of illness or disability. Not means-tested, but enough National Insurance contributions must have been paid in order to qualify. There is a short-term lower rate for the first 28 weeks of incapacity (if ineligible for statutory sick pay), a short-term higher rate from week 29 to week 52, and a long-term rate after 52 weeks.

11 Severe Disablement Allowance: this is a weekly cash benefit, tax-free and non-means-tested, for people who have been unable to work for at least 28 weeks but who do not have sufficient National Insurance contributions to qualify for incapacity benefit. It cannot normally be paid for the first time after the pensionable age. The regulations relating to this allowance are rather complicated, and it is advisable either to consult your local Social Security office or look at the comprehensive information given in the *Disability Rights Handbook.*

12 Hospital Patients' travelling expenses: this is available to both in-patients and out-patients, and although it is always available for those receiving family credit or income support, it can often apply to others on a fairly low income, and may cover the expenses of a friend or relative if an escort is needed (enquire at the hospital).

13 Tax allowances: these are described in the PAYE Coding Guide which comes with an income tax form, or is available from any Inland Revenue Office. Disabled people may be entitled to allowances such as the additional personal allowance for children where a wife is incapacitated, or to the daughter's service allowance where a daughter is caring for a parent. A reduction in Council Tax is also sometimes available for disabled people. Your local Council will be able to advise you about this.

14 Motability: this is a voluntary organisation which can help you to use your mobility allowance to get a car or electric wheelchair on terms better than you might otherwise obtain. A leaflet entitled 'Introducing Motability' is available from Social Security offices, and explains the scheme in detail.

Four key organisations

The Multiple Sclerosis Society

Headquarters: 25 Effie Road, Fulham,
London SW6 1EE
Tel. 0171–610 7171. Fax 0171–736 9861

MS Society Offices (Scotland) 0131–225 3600; (Northern Ireland) 01232 644914

MS Helpline (10 am–4 pm) 0171–371 8000

MS Counselling Lines – 24-hour service via referral from these answerphones: London 0171–222 3123; Midlands 0121–476 4229; Scotland 0131–226 6573

Much of the work of the Society and its branches has been described in Chapter 7, but it should be emphasised that for the MS sufferer the Society can offer much assistance on a variety of problems. Local branches can help through links with the Social Services, providing general advice, financial and practical help, and simply through contact with others who have faced or are facing the same problems. The details of local branches can be obtained from your local library, Citizens' Advice Bureau, telephone directory or, often, local newspaper.

The Disabled Living Foundation

380–384 Harrow Road, London W9 2HU
Tel. 0171–289 6111

The DLF provides a really valuable information service for the disabled and an aids centre. The information service can supply up-to-date information about manufacturers, stockists and prices on all of the daily living equipment on the market, whilst at the aids centre professional help and advice can be given, although it is wise to make an appointment in order to ensure that one of the advisers is available to help you.

The Disability Alliance ERA

1st Floor East, Universal House,
88–94 Wentworth Street, London E1 7SA
Tel. 0171–247 8776

This is a federation of sixty organisations of or for disabled people, with the aim of introducing a comprehensive approach to financing disability, and restructuring the existing methods of social security benefits. It publishes research reports on specific problems of disability and the *Disability Rights Handbook* encouraging the taking up of existing benefits, and also runs a *Welfare Rights Information Service* (telephone the *Rights Advice Line* on 0171–247 8763).

Royal Association for Disability and Rehabilitation (RADAR)

12 City Forum, 250 City Road,
London EC1V 8A7
Tel. 0171–250 3222

This is an important organisation, providing an information service for all aspects of disability. Its broadsheets of information on such subjects as employment, education, transport, wheelchairs and holidays are up to date and comprehensive. It also operates the National Key Scheme. For a small fee RADAR supplies a key and a list of 3000 accessible toilets. RADAR can also supply details of the twice-yearly excellent and independently organised NAIDEX Conference and Exhibition of aids and equipment.

Other agencies

Across Trust

Bridge House, 70–72 Bridge Road,
East Molesey, Surrey KT8 9HF
Tel. 0181–783 1355

Provides accompanied holidays for disabled people.

Association of Disabled Professionals

170 Benton Hill, Horbury,
West Yorkshire WF4 5HW
Tel. 01924 270335

Run by people with disabilities, providing advice on educational, rehabilitation, training and employment opportunities for the disabled. Maintains a Register of Professional Advisers who can offer advice on employment prospects in their particular fields and put people in touch with organisations and individuals who can help with educational and employment problems.

British Computer Society

1 Sansard Street,
Swindon, SN1 1HJ
Tel. 01793 480269

A specialist group which will offer specific advice on activities relating to computing and the disabled.

British Red Cross Society

9 Grosvenor Crescent,
London SW1X 7EJ
Tel. 0171–235 5454

Can often be helpful in solving problems of a practical nature, particularly with regard to transport or wheelchairs.

British Sports Association for the Disabled

Mary Glen Haig Suite,
Salecast House, 13–27 Brunswick Place,
London N1 6DX
Tel. 0171–490 4919

The recognised governing body for all types of sports for the disabled, obtaining grants for disabled sports and organising international sporting events.

Carers National Association

20–25 Glasshouse Yard,
London EC1A 4JS
Tel. 0171–490 8818

Offers a variety of support and information for carers, and can advise on and assist in setting up local self-help groups.

Continence Advisory Service

Dene Centre, Castle Farm Road,
Newcastle-upon-Tyne NE3 1PH
Tel. 0191 2130050 (Helpline)

Crossroads Care Attendance Schemes Ltd

10 Regent Place,
Rugby CV21 2PN
Tel. 01788 573653

Offers practical help for families with a disabled member.

DIG (Disablement Income Group)

Unit 5, Archway Business Centre,
19–23 Wedmore Street,
London N19 4RZ
Tel. 0171–263 3981

Provides a specialist advisory and information service concerning the financial welfare of disabled people and their families.

Disability Action (Northern Ireland)

2 Annadale Avenue, Belfast BT7 3JH
Tel. 01232 491011

Provides information and training services for people who are disabled, support to groups, advice on fund-raising and access. Also has a driving assessment centre and mobility information service and runs a placement scheme and employment service.

Disability Alliance ERA (see page 82)

Disability Law Service

Room 241, 49–51 Bedford Row,
London WC1R 4LR
Tel. 0171–831 8031

Offers free legal advice and information for disabled people.

Disability Scotland

Scottish Council on Disability, Princes House,
5 Shandwick Place, Edinburgh EH2 4RG
Tel. 0131–229 8632

Information service for the disabled in Scotland.

Disability Wales

Llys Ifor, Crescent Road,
Caerphilly, Mid Glamorgan CF8 1XL
Tel. 01222 887325

Information service for the disabled in Wales.

Disabled Access to Technology Association

Broomfield House, Bolling Road,
Bradford BD4 7BG
Tel. 01274 370019

Provides training in, for example, computing and business administration for disabled people.

Disabled Car Purchase

114 Commonwealth Road, Caterham,
Surrey CR3 6LS
Tel. 01883 345298

Supplies specialist vehicles.

Disabled Drivers' Association

Ashwellthorpe Hall, Ashwellthorpe,
Norwich NR16 1EX
Tel. 01508 489449

Will help and advise disabled people on all matters of mobility. An annual subscription entitles members to receive its magazine.

Disabled Drivers' Motor Club

Cosy Nook, Cottingham Way,
Thrapston, Northants NN14 4PL
Tel. 01832 734 724

Gives help and advice to the disabled motorist; the annual subscription entitles members to the Club's bi-monthly magazine.

Disabled Living Foundation (see page 82)

Federation of MS Therapy Centres

Unit 4, Murdock Road,
Bedford MK41 7PD
Tel. 01234 325781

Centres exist throughout the UK, providing a range of services including physiotherapy, oxygen therapy, counselling and dietary advice.

Gardening for Disabled Trust

Hayes Farmhouse, Hayes Lane,
Peasmarsh, East Sussex TN1 6XR

Provides information and advice on gardening; has a newsletter and garden club.

Gingerbread

16–17 Clerkenwell Close,
London E1R 0AA
Tel. 0171–336 8183

An association with over 370 local groups seeking to encourage and promote the interests of people who, for whatever reasons, have to support or care for their families alone. Group meetings are held and advisory literature is available.

Greater London Association of Disabled People

336 Brixton Road, London SW9 7AA
Tel. 0171–274 0107

Publishes monthly magazine *London Disability News* and other specialist publications. Aims to be a source of information on local and national welfare legislation, and to press for improvements in the quality of life for disabled Londoners.

Holiday Care Service

2nd Floor, Imperial Buildings, Victoria Road,
Horley, Surrey RH6 7PZ
Tel. 01293 774535

Will give advice and information about agencies to contact when arranging holidays for the disabled.

John Grooms Association for the Disabled

10 Gloucester Drive, London N4 2LP
Tel. 0181–802 7272

Provides care and accommodation for disabled people, running holiday hotels and self-catering holiday units. Through a housing association promotes provision of purpose-built flats for the disabled.

Leonard Cheshire Foundation

26–29 Maunsel Street, London SW1P 2QN
Tel. 0181–828 1822

Has 40 Family Support Services in England. The service offers part-time care attendants who can provide assistance in the home to people with a disability. Runs 75 residential homes for the disabled and provides some holiday accommodation. Provides a Special Care Agency to find help for disabled people with special needs living in their own home. The Foundation is non-profit making, and fees are kept to a minimum.

Mobility Centre, Banstead

Damson Way, Orchard Hill, Queen Mary's Avenue,
Carshalton, Surrey SM5 4NR
Tel. 0181–770 1151

Information and advice on any outdoor mobility problems, including provision of individual assessments and trial/demonstration facilities in relation to the choice of appropriate adaptations to wheelchair models. Enquiries should be made in writing.

Motability

2nd Floor, Gatehouse, West Gate, The High,
Harlow, Essex CM20 1HR
Tel. 01279 635666

An organisation that helps disabled people to obtain a vehicle or electric wheelchair using their higher rate mobility allowance within the Disability Living Allowance.

MS (Research) Charitable Trust

Spirella Building, Letchworth, Herts SG6 4ET
Tel. 01462 675613

Funds research and provides information on management of MS.

Multiple Sclerosis Resource Centre

4a Chapel Hill, Stanstead, Essex CM24 8AG
Tel. 01279 817101

Offers information and advice on MS.

Multiple Sclerosis Society (see page 81)

The Myelin Project

4 Cammo Walk, Edinburgh EH4 8AN
Tel. 0131 339 1316

International charity organisation funding research on remyelination.

National Bureau for Students with Disabilities (SKILL)

336 Brixton Road, London SW9 7AA
Tel. 0171–274 0565

Gives information on post-16 education for disabled people.

National Council for Voluntary Organisations

26 Bedford Square, London WC1B 3HU
Tel. 0171–636 4066

Issues helpful booklets on many subjects including a semi-annual directory called *Voluntary Agencies*, which lists all kinds of relevant organisations, with a brief description of the work of each.

National Listening Library

12 Lant Street, London SE1 1QH
Tel. 0171–407 9417

Offers a 'talking books' service for people who have difficulty reading.

National Mobility Centre, Mobility Information Service

Unit 2a, Atcham Industrial Estate, Shrewsbury SY4 4UG
Tel. 01743 761889

Offers information on mobility and driving assessments for disabled drivers. Also houses the *Disability Motorists' Federation*, which offers a planning service with maps showing wheelchair-friendly places, RADAR Key Scheme toilets etc. (call its MAPLINE on 01743 761181).

PHAB (Physically Handicapped and Able-bodied)

12–14 London Road,
Croydon CR0 2TA
Tel. 0181–667 9443

An organisation with the objective of integrating disabled and able-bodied people through leisure and social activities. Over 500 clubs meet regularly to share a variety of interests and activities, and some holiday residential courses are held each year in Britain.

REMAP

Hazeldene, Ightham,
Sevenoaks, Kent TN15 9AD
Tel. 01732 883818

Will make or adapt aids for disabled people when not available commercially.

Riding for the Disabled Association

Avenue R, National Agricultural Centre,
Kenilworth, Warwickshire CV8 2LY
Tel. 01203 696510

There are about 710 groups throughout the UK, each consisting of an organiser, secretary, riding instructor, usually a physiotherapist and other helpers. Occasionally riding is free but usually a small fee is payable. The book *Riding for the disabled* is available from the Association.

Royal Association for Disability and Rehabilitation (RADAR) (see page 83)

Queen Elizabeth's Foundation for the Disabled

Leatherhead Court, Woodland Road,
Leatherhead, Surrey KT22 0BN
Tel. 01372 842204

Comprises four units which provide assessment, further education, vocational training, residential sheltered work, holidays and convalescence for many hundreds of disabled people. Also has a resource centre and disabled information service.

SEQUAL

Ddol Hir, Glyn Ceiriog, Llangollen, Clwyd LL20 7NP
Tel. 01691 718331

Assists people with disabilities in finding suitable communication aids.

SPOD (Sexual Problems of the Disabled)

286 Camden Road, London N7 0BJ
Tel. 0171–607 8851

An organisation providing information and confidential advice on personal matters for people with disabilities. Holds a register of professional counsellors and publishes a series of informative leaflets. Also holds training courses.

Talking Newspapers

Heathfield, East Sussex TN21 8DB
Tel. 01435 866102

Puts people in touch with newspapers on cassette in their area.

Tripscope

The Courtyard, Evelyn Road,
London W4 5JL
Tel. 0181–994 9294

Travel information service for the disabled.

Some helpful reference books

The *Disability Rights Handbook*, a key publication, has already been discussed. Published each April, disabled people can purchase it at discount from the address given on page 82.

The *Multiple Sclerosis Society* supplies a range of publications, cassettes and videotapes on MS and related topics. See page 81 for address.

Further useful literature on disability issues is available from *RADAR* (address on page 83). In particular, RADAR has a number of helpful publications on access, mobility and employment for disabled people:

Access: A set of *Access Data Sheets* is available covering basic access information (e.g. width of doors, lifts, lavatories, access to buildings) extracted from the British Standard Code of Practice for Access for the Disabled to Buildings. RADAR also produces an access guide to the London underground and access guides, for example, to major cities such as London and Paris. Many towns and cities also have their own Access Guides available from Council or Tourist Information Offices. Books are also available from RADAR on access to Country Parks, Historic Buildings and general places of interest in the UK.

Mobility: In addition to a book entitled *Choosing a Wheelchair* and a number of *Mobility Fact Packs*, RADAR also produces, in conjunction with the Disabled Drivers' Motor Club, *The Disabled Motorist*, incorporating the *Disabled Motor Club Handbook*.

Employment: RADAR produces several publications on employment issues, including *Into Work: A guide for disabled people*; *Employment Rights: A guide for disabled people*; and a number of *Employment Fact Sheets*. It also has three fact sheets on the Disability Discrimination Act (1995), one of which deals with employment.

Notes

Chapter 1

1 See, for example, Matthews, W.B. (1993) *Multiple Sclerosis: The Facts*, 3rd edn (Oxford University Press) and Bauer, H.J. (1977) *A Manual on Multiple Sclerosis* (The International Federation of MS Societies). Also see the following articles: Burnfield, A. and Burnfield, P. (1978) 'Common Psychological Problems in Multiple Sclerosis', *British Medical Journal*, 1, 1193–4; Tallis, R.C. (1981) 'Multiple Sclerosis: Diagnosing MS and telling the patient', *MS News*, No. 107, Spring.

Chapter 2

1 Many sources have been drawn on for this chapter, the main books being Matthews, W.B. (1993) *Multiple Sclerosis: The Facts*; and Matthews, W.B., Compston, A., Allen, I.V. and Martyn, C.N. (1991) *McAlpine's Multiple Sclerosis*, Edinburgh, Churchill Livingstone.

2 Mumford, C.J. *et al.* (1994) 'The British Isles survey of multiple sclerosis in twins', *Neurology*, 44 (1), pp. 11–15.

3 Office of Population Censuses and Surveys (1995) *Morbidity Statistics from General Practice. Fourth National Study 1991/92*, London, HMSO.

4 Williams, E.S. and McKeran, R.O. (1986) 'Prevalence of multiple sclerosis in a South London borough', *British Medical Journal*, 293, pp. 237–9.

5 Robertson, N. and Compston, A. (1995) 'Surveying multiple sclerosis in the United Kingdom', *J. Neurology, Neurosurgery, and Psychiatry*, 58, pp. 2–6 (Editorial).

6 Compston, D.A.S. *et al.* (1995) 'Genes and susceptibility to multiple sclerosis', *Acta Neurologica Scandinavica*, Supplement 161, pp. 43–51.

7 Gale, C.R. and Martyn, C.N. (1995) 'Migrant studies in multiple sclerosis', *Progress in Neurobiology*, 47, pp. 425–48.

8 Mims, C. (1983) *MS News*, No. 117, Autumn, pp. 7–11.

9 See 'Does genetic engineering really hold the key?' *MS Insight*,

Supplement 1, Nov./Dec. 1995.

10 Loder, C. (1995) *Standing in the Sunshine*, London, Century.

11 'Interferon beta-1b in the treatment of multiple sclerosis: final outcome of the randomized controlled trial', *Neurology*, 1995, 45, pp. 1227–85.

12 These findings are impressive and seem likely to herald a new era in the treatment of MS. However, a note of caution should be sounded. Despite the effect of Betaferon in reducing the relapse rate in the treatment group, no significant differences were found in disability levels between the treatment and control groups at the end of the trial (i.e. the drug did not appear to limit progression of general disability in the MS patients). New drugs based on beta interferon 1a, on the other hand, may have the effect of reducing both relapse rates and the levels of physical disability associated with MS.

13 See Jacobs, L.D. *et al.* (1996) 'Intramuscular interferon beta-1a for disease progression in relapsing multiple sclerosis', *Annals of Neurology*, 39, 3, pp. 285–94.

14 It is also possible, of course, that the use of this expensive drug will be so severely rationed on financial grounds within some Health Authorities that a number of people with MS who are *clinically* appropriate cases for treatment will find that the treatment is not immediately available.

15 This treatment has also been found to be effective in another demyelinating disease which has some of the features of MS. This is the Guillain-Barre syndrome (GBS), which is the commonest cause of *acute* neuromuscular paralysis in the developed world today. As with MS, the Guillain-Barre syndrome is thought to result from some aberration in the body's immune response system. The prognosis of GBS is generally good, with about 80 per cent of patients making a full recovery.

16 Wiles, C.M. *et al.* (1986) 'Hyerbaric oxygen in multiple sclerosis: a double blind trial', *British Medical Journal*, 292, pp. 367–71.

17 Kleijnen, J. and Knipschild, P. (1995) 'Hyperbaric oxygen for multiple sclerosis. Review of controlled trials', *Acta Neurologica Scandinavica*, 91 (5), pp. 330–34.

18 Jones, R., Rees, D.P. and Campbell, M.J. (1991) 'EMG and force values during sustained contraction in MS patients – implications for therapy', in Wiethölter, H., Dichgans, J. and Mertin, J. (eds)

Current Concepts in Multiple Sclerosis, Excerpta Medica, Amsterdam.

Chapter 3

1 The MS Society provides a 24-hour counselling service and a Helpline for MS sufferers and their families or carers (see Chapter 7), and most MS branches offer some form of counselling advice.

2 SPOD (Sexual Problems of the Disabled), 286 Camden Road, London N7 0BJ. The MS Society also produces some helpful leaflets on sexual problems and multiple sclerosis.

3 *Recruiting and employing a personal care worker* is available from DIG (Disablement Income Group), Unit 5, Archway Business Centre, 19–23 Wedmore Street, London N19 4RZ. Tel. 0171–263 3981. Advice is also available from the Carers National Association (see Chapter 8).

Chapter 4

1 Burnfield, A. and Burnfield, P. (1978) (see note 1, Chapter 1).

2 There is even some evidence to suggest that the level of disease activity tends to *decrease* immediately following some surgical procedures and fractures.

3 Peace of Mind (Call Care Alert Unit), Communication Care Ltd, Communication House, 39 Invincible Road, Farnborough, Hampshire GU14 7QU. Tel. 01252 376746. AID-call Ltd, Linhay House, Ashburton, Devon TQ13 7UP. Tel. 01364 654321.

4 Details of these electronic systems can be obtained from:
Possum Controls Ltd, Unit 8, Farmbrough Close, Aylesbury Vale Industrial Park, Stocklake, Aylesbury, Bucks HP20 1DQ. Tel. 01296 81591.
and
Hugh Steeper Ltd, Queen Mary's University Hospital, Roehampton Lane, London SW15 5PL. Tel. 0181–788 0137.

Chapter 5

1 Obtained from Metco Walkabouts, 17 Ireton Grove, Attenborough, Nottingham NG9 6BJ. Tel. 01159 255488.

2 Available from Uniscan Ltd, 38 Hornsby Square, Southfields Industrial Estate, Laindon, Basildon, Essex SS15 6SD. Tel. 01268 419288.

3 The Buggy Major is available from Andrew Mclaren Ltd, Station Works, Long Buckby, Northampton NN6 7PF. Tel. 01327 842662.

4 This allowance can of course be paid directly into a bank or building society account.

5 From Cunningham, D.J. (1977) *Stigma and social isolation: self-perceived problems of a group of multiple sclerosis sufferers.* Health Services Research Unit, University of Kent at Canterbury.

6 The Act also requires that unless there is good reason employers should not treat a disabled person less favourably than someone else because of their disability, a stipulation that applies to all employment matters including recruitment, training, promotion and dismissal.

7 *Holidays in the British Isles: a guide for disabled people* and *European holidays and travel abroad: a guide for disabled people* are published by RADAR, 12 City Forum, 250 City Road, London EC1V 8A7. A set of *Holiday Fact Packs* is also available.

8 *The National Key Scheme: accessible toilets for disabled people* is published by RADAR (see note 7 above).

9 *Care in the air.* From Air Transport Users Committee, 129 Kingsway, London WC2B 6NN.

10 Cloet, A. and Underhill, C. (1982) *Gardening is for everyone* Souvenir Press.

11 Leaflets on bird watching for the disabled can be obtained free of charge from RSPB, The Lodge, Sandy, Bedfordshire SG19 2DL. Tel. 01767 680551.

Chapter 6

1 *How to keep your cholesterol in check* by Robert Povey.

2 At the moment the role of linoleic acid in our bodies is not fully understood, and the precise clinical significance of this finding has yet to be determined. However, there is some evidence, discussed later in this chapter, that a diet high in linoleic acid may be of benefit to people with MS.

3 From the linoleic acid obtained from such sources our bodies can then produce other omega-6 fatty acids such as arichidonic acid (also found in small quantities in meat) and gamma linolenic acid or GLA (also found in evening primrose and borage oils).

4 Dworkin, R.H., Bates, D., Millar, J.H.D. and Paty, D.W. (1984) 'Linoleic acid and multiple sclerosis: a reanalysis of three double blind trials', *Neurology*, 34, pp. 1441–5.

5 In general, nutritionists advise that it is much better to concentrate on obtaining such vitamins by eating a variety of foods in which they are contained, rather than by taking vitamin supplements.

6 The importance of actively involving people with movement disorders in finding ways of overcoming their own particular problems is also stressed in an approach, originally developed in Hungary, called Conductive Education. Its main use has been with children having cerebral palsy, but there has also been some work with adults suffering from neurological disorders such as Parkinson's Disease and MS. For details contact: The Foundation for Conductive Education, The National Institute of Conductive Education, Cannon Hill House, Russell Road, Moseley, Birmingham B13 8RD. Tel. 0121–449 1569.

7 A useful organisation is *Yoga for Health Foundation*, Ickwell Bury, Northill, Biggleswade, Bedfordshire SG18 9ES. Tel. 01767 627271. It arranges day courses and 5-day residential courses for people with MS.

8 What happens is that our bodies need vitamin D in order to absorb calcium, and apart from a few foods which contain the vitamin (like fish oils and some margarines), this vitamin is made by the body using sunlight.

9 Your physiotherapist or local pain clinic will be able to advise you about the purchase of a suitable TENS machine.

Chapter 8

1 The provisions of the Act have been reinforced by the Disabled Persons (Services, Consultation and Representation) Act (1986) and other Community Care legislation. Under these, local authorities are required, for example, to assess people's needs for services (including those of school-leavers with disabilities); to provide people with as much relevant information as possible; to take carers' abilities into account when undertaking an assessment; and to ensure that adequate help is available to the disabled person.

2 For full reference see note 4 for Chapter 4.

3 See note 7 for Chapter 5.

Index